D0018347

Food Allergy Field Guide
A Lifestyle Manual for Families

What People Are Saying About.....
Food Allergy Field Guide

According to recent research, gluten sensitivity is now being recognized as a common rather than rare disease, and is often accompanied by other immunologic food sensitivities. Thus, a very large portion of the American population will need to be made aware of the health risks posed by common everyday foods. Ms. Willingham's book is an excellent starting place for those individuals and/or families who have been diagnosed with gluten or other food sensitivities, or who care enough about their health to prevent such reactions. The tips on how children can eat to their health specifications without appearing "different' are especially useful. This book will be a welcome addition to references recommended by health care professionals to their food-sensitive patients. —**Kenneth Fine, M.D., Intestinal Health Institute, FinerHealth and Nutrition**

Breezy, uplifting, yet "meaty" and informative.—**Nancy Carol Sanker, OTR, Director of Educational Support Groups, Asthma and Allergy Foundation of America**

As assistant to the director at a nursery school, I am involved in both alerting teachers about allergies and the preparation of non-allergenic snacks, if applicable, for the children. I know from personal experience that it is very important to pay attention to allergies from a health standpoint, demonstration of cooperation and communication with parents, and also giving children the best opportunity to learn without food-related behavioral side effects. This new resource for families with children with food sensitiveities is a valuable, sensible asset for those families with children who have either food intolerance and/or allergies. Very often people with one food sensitivity seem to develop problems with others. This resource gives specific coping information in terms of lifestyle suggestions, dietary substitutions, personal stories, recipes, and other resources in order to empower the family and the child to live as normal and healthy as possible. Each chapter's summary and the Appendix give details about sensitivity to wheat, dairy, peanuts, eggs, corn, and soy. I certainly agree with one main goal of this resource, which is to help your child 'eat differently without feeling different.'—**Janet Y. Rinehart, Chairman, Houston Celiac Sprue Support Group, Past President, CSA/USA, Inc.**

Food Allergy Field Guide
A Lifestyle Manual for Families

Savory Palate, Inc.
8174 S. Holly, # 404
Littleton, CO 80122-4004
www.savorypalate.com

Copyright ©2000 by Theresa Willingham

Library of Congress Card Number: 00-105115
ISBN 1-889374-07-5
Printed in the United States of America

First Edition, 2000

SUMMARY
1. Wheat-free, gluten-free, celiac, cookbook, autism
2. Wheat intolerance, gluten intolerance, food sensitivity, food allergy

Edited by Mary Bonner
Cover design by Shaeffer Reagan Design

For information, contact:
Savory Palate, Inc.
8174 South Holly, #404   www.savorypalate.com
Littleton, CO, 80122-4004 (800) 741-5418   (303) 741-5408

CONTENTS

Part III
Eat, Drink, and Be Merry:
Cooking for Health and Happiness

Acknowledgements

A book this comprehensive could not have been written without the moral, intellectual, and professional support and inspiration of many individuals and organizations.

Principal among these are the families who so generously shared their tribulations and their triumphs, their hindsight and their insights in an effort to help those coming after them. So it is with deep gratitude and heartfelt appreciation for their time and effort that I acknowledge the following families: Amadeos, Benkofskes, Bulmers, Dowdles, Faulhabers, Korns, Sawyers, Seebaurs, Thomases, Winfreys, and Wolfskills; and these individuals: "Cindy," "Edith," and "Sharon."

And many thanks to the children who lent their experiences and insights to this book, whose voices—like the voices of all children—deserve to be heard in matters that concern them and whose experiences and feelings—like the experiences and feelings of all children—deserve to be honored. Thank you *very much* Jessica, Jimmy, Joshua, Miri, Nathan, Nicole, and Tyler.

I also want to thank Linda Blanchard, who shared family experiences and professional resources with her "No Milk" page; Dr. Joan Fleitas with her wonderful "Bandaides and Blackboards" website; Nigel Dobson-Keeffe, who also shared his own experiences as well as his wonderful website, "Milk Allergy and Lactose Intolerance;" Audrey Kinsella for her assistance, encouragement, and support; Steve Kinsley, of Nu Connexions software who shared resources and insights; Katherine Murray for sharing her experiences, and the resources on her "Children with Milk, Egg, and Other Food Allergies" page; Dr. Harris Steinman, with his wonderful FAP AID database who shared so generously of his All Allergy Net site and demo software; and Melissa Taylor of Food Allergy Survivors Together (FAST), who has become a fast friend, as well.

And a special thank you to my friends: Lorraine, for talking food without end, with laughter, joy, and love; Shelly, whose friendship makes all things possible; and Jan, who always warms my heart and soul. Thank you all so very much. And a very special thank you to Carol Fenster, of Savory Palate, Inc., without whose kind mentoring, support, and encouragement, this book would never have seen the light of day.

Several experts also contributed to this book: Kenneth Fine, M.D., Intestinal Health Institute, Dallas, TX; Ed Hoffenberg, M.D. and Amy Andersen Drescher, R.D., of The Children's Hospital, University of Colorado Health Sciences Center; John M. James, Colorado Allergy & Asthma Centers, P.C.; Janet Y. Rinehart, Past President CSA/USA and current president, Houston Celiac Sprue Support Group; Cynthia Kupper, R.D., Gluten Intolerance Group of NA; Ellen Speare, Certified Nutritionist, Wild Oats Markets; Nancy Carol Sanker, OTR, Asthma and Allergy Foundation of America; Peggy Wagener, Sully's Living Without; Mary K. Sharrett, M.S., R.D., Children's Hospital, Columbus, OH; Martha Steffen, P.A.-C, Colorado Allergy & Asthma Centers; Debbie Lee, Nutritionist, and Sue Wielgopolan and Denise Roth—mothers of celiac children.

And while it goes without saying, not to say it would be a terrible omission: A book like this could also not have been written without the support, patience, encouragement, and love of my family. Thank you Steven, my husband, best friend, and live-in editor, for your indulgence and never-ending faith in me. Thank you Elizabeth and Andrea, my two very patient daughters who often helped with secretarial duties and impromptu backrubs. And thank you, Chris, my special inspiration for this book, whose endless good nature and happy contributions to my life and to the lives of those around him are reason enough to eat well, live well, and be happy.

Thank you one and all, for making this book possible.

"In good health", *Theresa Willingham*

Introduction

*I am not a doctor, nor do I play one on TV. I am the mother of a child who cannot eat wheat. The information presented in **The Food Allergy Field Guide** is the result of my own research and experiences, and that of the shared experiences of several other families, for whose help and generosity I am truly grateful. All children are individuals and all conditions can manifest themselves differently.*

This is a dietary and lifestyle guide, not a medical book, *even though some general medical information is discussed. I cannot suggest strongly enough that you and your child work with a good pediatric gastroenterologist or allergist for definitive medical advice and assistance, or at least have access to physicians, nutritionists, dietitians, and medical facilities that are knowledgeable about food sensitivities.*

Chris' Story

He weighed more than 9 lbs. when he was born, robust, ruddy, and squalling; the picture of health. My new son, our third child, had a head of dark hair, big compelling eyes, and a strong, gregarious personality that, by four months of age, was captivatingly obvious. His smiling eyes and engaging sense of humor charmed everyone.

He was also a messy, noisy, squirming feeder and, with two other young children to care for, it was difficult to nurse him patiently. When Chris was around six or seven months old, I started supplementing him with formula, with the doctor's okay and my own experience to reassure me—and I failed to make the connection when he started having digestive problems.

He had chronic diaper rashes that I fought daily to control, and noisy, gassy, and frequent bowel movements. And yet he

1

thrived, never got colds or fevers, and was endlessly good-natured. It was a dichotomy that would puzzle me for more than two years. Putting him on solid foods didn't seem to help at all, even though he was a voracious eater and scarfed down Cheerios™ like a vacuum cleaner!

It wasn't until I was leafing half-heartedly through a medical book, wondering vaguely what I was looking for, that I came across a description of celiac disease, a type of wheat sensitivity. I stopped. I stared. I read the passage a half dozen times. Then I snatched away the Cheerios™. The medical description of this food sensitivity—a reaction to the protein in wheat—described Chris to a T, and the Cheerios™ weren't helping anything. In fact, they were part of the problem.

Now, to be honest, I had heard of wheat intolerance before, and had even fleetingly considered it our culprit as early as his first birthday, but I discounted it just as quickly for some reason and gave him his big, wheaty birthday cake as planned. Now there was no denying it. All the symptoms of this "rare" wheat sensitivity fit:

  • Bowel movements immediately after eating that were
      loose, floating, and difficult to flush away, along with
  • Bloating, and little weight gain.

Sometimes developmental delays were associated with the disorder, and while it was nothing conclusive, Chris had, indeed, been slow to walk (although he was an aggressive and headlong crawler!) and at 2 ½, was stuttering badly when he talked. He was quite tall, but very slender with the "wasted buttocks" look often associated with celiac disease. There was no way to tell if any of these things, or the myriad unsettling suspicions I'd long entertained were, in reality, connected. But there was one way I could find out if wheat was, indeed, the problem.

2

The Trial Diet

I began to keep a journal of what Chris ate, when his bowel movements occurred, and what they looked like. When I voiced my suspicions to a friend and told her what I was doing, she looked at me dubiously. Evidently I looked somewhat obsessive documenting my toddler's bathroom habits. But, like any scientific endeavor, one needs to know the facts before one can draw any conclusions. And I was determined to know the facts.

At the same time I started the dietary journal, I began scouring the Internet for information about wheat sensitivities and came across a very informative article that suggested eliminating wheat from the diet for six weeks, and keeping a record of the results. My record keeping was vindicated! We eliminated the wheat and in little more than a week's time, Chris's bowel movements had gone from more than four a day, to just two or three. In two weeks, he became slightly constipated, which was a real switch. After six weeks, his symptoms had almost completely cleared and we headed to the doctor with our findings.

The doctor concurred with our findings and agreed that Chris appeared to be sensitive to wheat. She said she would have recommended the same course of action to test our suspicions (had she thought of it!) and told us we could continue with the wheat-free diet, which wouldn't hurt him and obviously relieved the symptoms. Or, she said, we could verify our suspicions more precisely with a biopsy, the only way to definitively diagnose celiac disease—which his wheat sensitivity resembled.

Because of his age and the success of the relatively simple treatment, we opted to stay with the diet, especially since there is yet no cure for celiac disease. Nor is there a cure for lactose intolerance, or cow milk allergy, or corn or rice sensitivities or the myriad other food sensitivities that, according to the Centers for Disease Control, afflict up to 6% of children under the age of three.

I Was Not Alone

As I struggled to get a handle on Chris's problems, other parents around the world were struggling with their children's food sensitivities. Lindsay[1] agonized over her 14-month-old son's constant, projectile vomiting and a rash that wouldn't go away, unconvinced by her pediatrician's reassurance that these events were "normal." Her son has celiac disease.

Karen's son stopped gaining weight after the age of one and seemed to have an inordinate number of bowel movements each day. He, too, has celiac disease.

Sharon's daughter became wheezy and congested sometimes after meals, a problem that cleared up as soon as her egg sensitivity was identified.

Katherine was stumped by her daughter's incontinence and gas pains, and found both stopped after she took milk out of her diet. Others dealt with behavioral problems, short stature, failure to thrive, or autism which was worsened by certain foods.

And all were making the same fundamental discovery: there's no substitute for parents when it comes to both learning about and handling food sensitivities in children. No one is as interested in our children as we are. Frequently, parents find that well-meaning doctors label food sensitivity symptoms as "common" colic, or ear infections, or viruses. Antibiotics are prescribed when wheat should be withheld. Colic drops are offered when milk may be the culprit. Parents who take charge, who take the time to become educated about their children's medical conditions, can take justifiable pride when they discover their child's chronic diarrhea is the result of a food sensitivity and not

---

[1] For privacy reasons, only first names are used in case discussions.

4

a never-ending virus, or that their jittery, chronically distracted child finds focus with a change of diet.

But once that discovery is made, that's where the adventure really begins. Feeding a toddler fruits and vegetables is relatively easy. Helping young children negotiate the maze of birthday parties, restaurant outings, vacations, picnics, and everything else an ordinary kid[2] encounters, in addition to feeding other unafflicted members of the family, requires a little more thought and planning. And that's what this book is all about: *How to live with a food-sensitive child so that you, your child, and the rest of the family can live rewarding, healthy, and happy lives.*

A Field Guide For Life

This is not a cookbook—although you'll find many really good recipes here. And it's not a medical book. This is a lifestyle

book, because kids deserve enjoyable lifestyles and because life, with or without a food sensitivity, is worth living well and meaningfully.

> *"Most of the time it doesn't bother me very much that I can't have wheat. There's a lot of other stuff that I can eat, like rice and beans, and fruit—especially bananas. I like bananas!—and Jell-O™ and corn chips and tacos and some kinds of hot dogs (with no buns) and jellybeans! My favorite thing to eat is the rice flour pancakes my mom makes. I also like Cocoa Blasts™ and Corn Pops™. I never go hungry."*—Chris, 7.

I'm calling this a *field guide* because like any good, user-friendly reference book, it's designed to be a comprehensive, thorough identification guide and resource manual. When you're out in the "field" of life with your food sensitive child, shopping, eating out, going to parties or picnics, camping out or cooking in, you need to know your way around. You need to be able to identify friends

---

[2] To avoid gender bias (and the bulkiness of using "they" or "their" or s/he), we're going to be using "he" and "she" interchangeably throughout, but all of the issues we'll discuss apply equally to boys and girls.

5

and foes, sanctuaries and sink holes, the edible and the inedible. This is your field guide to the good life for your food-sensitive child.

Healthy Birthrights
The first step towards that lifestyle is the knowledge that a food sensitivity isn't the end of the world. As a matter of fact, food sensitivities like celiac disease and lactose intolerance and cow milk allergy can be cloaking a healthy birthright that obligates your child to a diet most Americans would do well to emulate—pure, fresh foods, untainted by preservatives or additives.

What I offer you here is practical, everyday guidance to help both you and your food-sensitive children live that kind of life, too. The goal of this "field guide" is to teach you and your children to deal with their special dietary needs on a daily basis without compromising their childhood or that of their siblings. The trick, for children, is *eating differently without seeming different.*

The field guide will also help empower food-sensitive children, using tips and insights from children just like themselves who have found that a diet that doesn't make them sick shouldn't make them seem different, either.

> *"If you're allergic to wheat, don't be upset or sad because it's okay. If you go to parties, you can always eat corn chips and sherbet and on your birthday, your mom can make you a wheat-free cake or a Jello® cake. My mom made me a Jello® cake once. She put whipped cream on it and made it look like a lifesaver. It also looked a little like a flower. Sometimes people offer me stuff I can't have, and I just tell them I'm allergic to wheat."—Chris, 7*

As Chris himself will tell you, "I can't eat wheat, but I like to have fun." So let the fun begin!

6

Part I:
The World of Food Sensitivities

Chapter I
The Food Sensitive Toddler:
"No Cheerios™ for me, please."

Cheerios™, or some similar round, stubby-finger, friendly type of crunchy oat and wheat cereal has become a staple food for toddlers. And with good reason: they're healthy and whole-some, fairly easy to vacuum up, and the dog can safely eat the ones that fall under the table. We took them everywhere when my girls were little. In little plastic boxes or sealed bags, to snack on in waiting lines, at the beach––anywhere we needed an easy, portable time and attention filler. They were great; and my little boy loved them, too.

So it was with some sadness that I took them out of the family diet when I found out Chris was sensitive to wheat. Cheerios™ and I went back a long way and I felt like I was losing an old friend. Same for the slices of bread I would nonchalantly hand a hungry child who just couldn't wait for dinner; and zwieback teething toast, and crackers and muffins and cupcakes and cookies and hotdogs and hamburgers in toasted buns and all the other wonderful, wheaty foods that define American childhood. Convenience, I was convinced, was dead.

At the same time, I had no intention of continuing to subject Chris to the bloated, gassy bouts of chronic diarrhea he suffered at the hands of Cheerios™[3] and its brethren.

The same eye-opening dietary epiphany affects those who

---

[3] While Cheerios™ are largely composed of oats, a controversial grain for celiacs, the malt in this grain is also a culprit to the wheat sensitive.

7

would just as routinely hand their lactose intolerant or milk-allergic baby a bottle of milk or little cubes of cheese. You are suddenly thrust out of the ordinary and routine world of babyhood. You can't let your child share in playgroup snacks or playground picnics. Your baby can't slather ice cream all over her face at a birthday party. The long and the short of a food sensitivity is this: *Your child can't tolerate what your neighbors and all of your friends feed their toddlers. Even before your child can begin to feel different—YOU feel different.*

But it's important to put things in perspective and the best way to do that is to understand the mechanisms behind food sensitivities. The Asthma and Allergy Foundation (AAFA) estimates that as many as 50 million Americans suffer from some type of allergy, and of these, anywhere from 5% to 10% are believed to be food-related sensitivities.[4] But it's often difficult to distinguish between true food allergies and other reactions to food.

Allergy or Intolerance?
Although some experts disagree on the definition of allergies versus intolerances, the term "food intolerance"[5] is typically used to describe reactions to food that do not involve the immune system. These types of reactions include malabsorption problems due to enzyme deficiencies such as lactose intolerance, reactions to naturally occurring chemicals in foods such as salicylates in fruit, reactions to food contaminants such as bacteria, and reactions to preservatives such as sulfites,

---

4 Snyder, O.P. and D. M. Poland, "Adverse Reactions to Food, Food Allergy and Sensitivity: A Retail Food Hazard Problem," Hospitality Institute of Technology and Management, St. Paul, Minnesota, June, 1997. Also, see AAFA's "Get A Jump on Asthma and Allergies" brochure <www.aafa.org/getajump>.

5 "The Basics of Food Allergy and Intolerance," National Institute of Allergy and Infectious Diseases, National Institutes of Health, Date Published: January 1999. Date Reviewed: Nov. 16, 1999

flavorings such as monosodium glutamate, and colorants such as tartrazine.

True "allergic" reactions to food typically involve immediate immunological responses (hypersensitivity (IgE) and delayed T-cell mediated responses (non-IgE) to certain foods, and may occur from very small amounts of the food that triggers the response. The reaction can be as severe as anaphylaxis, which is characterized by shortness of breath, drop in blood pressure, and loss of consciousness, or as uncomfortable as gastrointestinal distress like nausea, vomiting, headaches, hives, and rashes. Allergic reactions to food can occur immediately or up to many hours or days after ingesting the offending food or ingredient.

To further complicate things, "food intolerance" and "food allergy" are often used—with debatable accuracy—almost interchangeably. But—'nuff said! It's confusing, but food sensitivities—the term *we're* going to use—can be like that.

What you need to know is what foods make your child feel badly, fail to thrive or create behavioral or learning problems, and what foods don't. Let the doctors work out the technical details.[6] We'll work on the practical ones.

The foods considered most likely to cause reactions in sensitive people are eggs, cow milk, peanuts, legumes, seafood, corn, wheat and related grains like barley and rye,[7] and tree nuts.[8]

---

[6] Dr. William G. Crook, an internationally recognized pediatrician, also believes that yeast is a contributing factor in food sensitivities and some childhood conditions such as ear problems, attention deficit hyperactivity disorder, and autism. He feels a particular strain of yeast, candida, is responsible. Although a discussion of this relationship is beyond our scope here, you may wish to visit Dr. Crook's web site at www.candida-yeast.com

[7] Until recently, oats were always included in this list. More on oats in subsequent chapters. See also Hoffenberg, Ed, M.D., et al., in press, Journal of Pediatrics.

8 Snyder, "Adverse Reactions to Food, Food Allergy and Sensitivity: A Retail Food Hazard Problem."

9

The Trouble with Diagnosis

While the effects of dietary changes can be far reaching for children, getting a proper diagnosis can be difficult. The fact that the symptoms of these food sensitivities so often mimic common childhood ailments—and that so many doctors are unfamiliar with celiac disease or unwilling to believe a baby might be sensitive to milk or wheat or other foods—makes it particularly difficult to pinpoint some of these food sensitivities in very young children.

Lindsay's Story

Lindsay's son, Sam, endured nine months of recurring ear infections that began when he was seven months old. "At thirteen months, he started having loose stools," said Lindsay. "They progressively got worse until by fifteen months they would run down his legs and out of the highchair to splash on the floor. The volume was incredible. They were mustard-yellow stools I now recognize as celiac stools and had a terrible odor. He cried constantly and wanted to be held."

Sam was also suffering from what Lindsay described as "strange, projectile type vomiting" and "a rash no one could diagnose." She says, "All during this…our pediatrician kept saying, 'Kids get diarrhea, don't worry.' And 'It's either the ear infections or the antibiotics.' But I was starting to get really scared."

Lindsay finally turned to an allergist, making the logical assumption that "with diarrhea, vomiting and a rash, Sam's body was trying desperately to get rid of something." Unfortunately, celiac disease doesn't show up on the regular "skin prick" tests allergy physicians commonly use to diagnose allergic reactions, and that doctor couldn't find what was wrong either.

10

Lindsay was saddened and frustrated by the same dead-end diagnosis wall thousands of other parents come up against with celiac disease and other food sensitivities. "The lack of help I was getting with a diagnosis made me feel very alone in finding out what was wrong," she recalled. "I am an assertive person, but I didn't know where to turn to get an answer when all results were coming up negative."

She pointed out to her son's pediatrician that he had lost 25% of his body weight in three months, and demanded stool and blood tests. When they, too, came up negative, she turned to another pediatrician who—on her first visit—said her son had a malabsorption problem and ran a celiac blood screen along with some other tests. A biopsy the following week confirmed that Sam had celiac disease. Lindsay finally had some answers and Sam was finally on his way to good health.

Lynda's Story
Lynda went through a similarly grueling period with her son Nathan. "Nathan pretty much stopped gaining weight after he turned one," she recalled. She said she asked the doctor, "Why does Nathan have such a big stomach? Why does he poop so much (three to four times a day)?" She was told, 'Don't worry, that's normal.'

"When Nathan was 21 months old, he started getting sick— really bad diarrhea, tired, throwing up sometimes. For a month, he was at the doctor every week. At first they thought it was the flu, then maybe giardia. After about a month of not getting better—actually getting much worse as by now he was throwing up every day, many diarrheas a day, no energy and he went from 26 lbs. to 21 lbs.—I demanded something be done."

Nathan was admitted to the hospital and tested for parasitic infections and cystic fibrosis. After three days with no results, Nathan's parents insisted on transferring him to a children's

11

hospital. Nathan was admitted to Minneapolis Children's Hospital where his parents met with a pediatric gastroenterologist who did some blood work and ran a biopsy. The results of both the blood work and the biopsy proved that Nathan had celiac disease. "From the day Nathan was diagnosed and started eating gluten free, he has not thrown up," says Lynda with satisfaction.

Danna's Story

Eight years ago, Danna Korn, who now runs an international celiac support group called R.O.C.K (Raising Our Celiac Kids) in San Diego County, CA and recently authored a book on the subject, [9] went through three doctors trying to find out what was wrong with her son, Tyler.

"Tyler was nine months old when he developed chronic diarrhea. He went through up to 22 diapers a day, and the doctors were telling me not to worry; diarrhea is difficult to get rid of once it starts. They attributed it to the flu, a virus, antibiotics (for frequent earaches). I switched doctors four times. The first three said nothing was wrong, especially because he was still in the 75th percentile for weight. It wasn't until nine months after the diarrhea started that I finally ended up with doctor number four. By this time, Tyler looked like a Biafra baby—extremely large, distended belly, skinny arms and legs, no energy whatsoever."

Tyler's fourth doctor agreed with Danna that something was very wrong and referred them to a pediatric gastroenterologist who tested Tyler for cancer, cystic fibrosis, and other ailments. Finally, they ran a biopsy. "This was in 1990. The standard was to do a biopsy, then go gluten free, do a second biopsy, then

---

[9]Korn, Danna, Kids with Celiac Disease: A Family Guide to Raising Happy, Healthy Gluten-Free Kids , Woodbine House, 2001.

challenge and follow-up with a third. That was the course we took, and he was diagnosed as being celiac."

Barbara's Story

"My son seemed to have a cold from birth," recalled Barbara. "The pediatrician treated him for those symptoms and finally pneumonia (in the summer). When he was six months old, we switched pediatricians, and the new one noticed the little scabs on his forehead. We thought he always just scratched himself. She predicted he was trying to relive the itching from an allergy. I was still breast feeding him, and her prediction that he had a milk allergy was right on target." It also turned out that her son was sensitive to wheat, eggs, and caffeine, as well.

But identifying the problem is only the first step. The next step is accepting the fact that your child will, most likely, have to eat a special diet for life. And that takes commitment from both of you. And that, I know, can be easier said than done—especially if you've got a picky eater on your hands.

The Picky Eater

Actually, I can't offer much advice to those who may have fussy eaters except this: A matter-of-fact treatment towards all good food—without using food as rewards or bargaining chips —goes a long way towards making good eaters.

My oldest daughter, who definitely has the finicky food gene in the family, just has to make do when we serve foods she doesn't care for. Interestingly enough, because we never made a big deal out of her recalcitrance to try new foods when she was younger, she has grown into a far more accepting and well-rounded eater than we would have predicted.

Lindsay approaches the food issue as routinely as possible, too. "Although we basically eat gluten free at home because it is easier to cook one meal, the rest of the family eats their own

13

bread, pasta and cereal. I am very careful not to make a big deal out of food and we never comment on how good our bread or dessert is. I also don't make anything special that is not gluten free, which is why my husband and I both had gluten-free birthday cakes since the dessert is the focus of attention.

We just tell Sam 'that is not for you, here is your X' (which I always make sure is something he loves) and 'that has gluten, it will make your tummy hurt'. The developmental issues of raising a child with a chronic illness are more important to me than just managing the diet. Most of all, I try to watch Sam and keep up with his cues. If he doesn't care that his food doesn't match, why should I?"

So if your food-sensitive toddler insists on bread and Cheerios™ (or whatever food he can't have) and won't eat anything else, sit next to him and munch on something safe for a while. Eventually, hunger and curiosity will probably win him over. If it doesn't, you'll need another book on that subject.

We'll just proceed with the hopeful assumption that your child will do anything for a comfortable, happy tummy or is old enough to know what's good for him and is willing to comply. Your job is to make it easy and casual, so it's routine for life.

> *"I remember not having enough energy to do the things normal kids could do, though I didn't know at the time why that was. I was always sick. There would be times when I had to lay perfectly still on the couch so I wouldn't vomit. But once I did I had to make a beeline to the bathroom. That was when I was about eight or nine. I also remember my mom's bran muffins that I loved always made me feel terrible."*
> —Jessica, now 16

Starting Fresh
With a toddler, that starts with simply replacing what was *routine* with what's *allowed*. That means ditch the Cheerios™,

and the teething toast for the wheat-sensitive kid and the cheese and ice cream for the one who can't have dairy products.

While you don't have to rely exclusively on health food items for your child's special diet, the health food store is a good place to go to start finding out what's available for babies and toddlers with sensitive tummies. Rice crackers are the easiest substitute for crunchy crackers. And puffed corn and rice cereals are the new finger food. Read ingredient labels carefully.

The fewer the ingredients—and the more recognizable—the better. If your child is gluten sensitive, be aware that seemingly benign things like hydrolyzed vegetable protein may contain wheat gluten. If your child can't have corn, be diligent about flavorings and things like caramel coloring, which is often made from corn. However, caramel coloring is gluten free.

Familiarize yourself with the many products offered in health food stores. Many health food stores also offer cooking classes that show you how to cook without wheat, milk, eggs, or other allergens. As time goes on, you'll be able to apply your new knowledge to the health food section of your local grocery store. Many grocery stores are becoming more health-food conscious and are carrying a wider selection of products for food-sensitive individuals.

For the wheat sensitive, there are a lot of generally available brands that are adaptable to special diets. Many Arrowhead Mills® bag cereals, for instance, are perfectly acceptable in place of more expensive brands and available at almost any grocery store. The old reliable Corn Pops™ cereal is inexpensive and fits the gluten-free bill, as well as having the added advantage of not crushing easily and thus making a great portable snack. So is Quaker Oats Cocoa Blasts™, which Chris came to love as a snack food (no oat products here, despite the brand name). We're pretty fond of them, too, as a matter of fact.

15

After a while, we found that Chris was checking the boxes as carefully as we were. "No wheat?" he would ask seriously. "No wheat" we would assure him, and he'd dig in.

And there's a huge line of products available in the dairy food section of many stores for lactose and cow-milk-allergy folks. There are dairy-free products from cheeses to milk. There are also egg-substitute products, and many products now carry labels warning of peanuts or other nut ingredients for individuals suffering sensitivities to these foods. Of course, the most important thing you can do, as you sort through the wealth of available alternatives, is to ALWAYS read the labels. Some of those "dairy-free" products can still have something like "sodium caseinate" in them, which is derived from casein. But it's definitely not the task it was even a few years ago to go gluten or dairy-free, or to avoid other problem foods.

There are entire websites devoted to food sensitivities, as well as a myriad of companies that sell "special diet" foods and countless "allergy-free" recipe books (see Appendix). There are also some excellent shopping guides to help you negotiate the grocery store aisles. Browse the web, look on your library bookshelves, and you'll find you are definitely not alone! The only thing consistently lacking, it seems, is a single reliable resource bringing it all together—and that's what I'm going to try to give you here.

KISS: Keep it Simple and Safe

Remember that most of what you need you'll find right on your local grocery shelves or growing on trees and vines. For toddlers and preschoolers, it's relatively easy to come up with safe munchies, whatever the sensitivity. For the over-three crowd with wheat sensitivities, raisins, nuts, seeds, popcorn, corn chips, corn nuts, cheese, and most canned fruits are fine. Rice crackers spread with peanut butter (or a nut butter substitute)

16

make a great snack, as do dried fruits, and cut up vegetables like carrot sticks and celery.

For the milk-free toddlers, almost all the same snacks can be used, but obviously avoid cheeses. Those with egg sensitivities do fine on the pure and wholesome stuff, too. And the same with nut sensitivities: the fewer ingredients in what you feed your child, the better.

Now... a note about rice crackers before we go much further. As easy and tasty and convenient as they are, excessive consumption of any one alternative grain—particularly in as easily a digestible form as the rice cracker—can trigger new sensitivities to the alternative grain. So, relying too heavily on rice could—and has been known to—create a sensitivity to rice which can definitely put a damper on things by taking one more selection out of your child's diet. The key to any healthy diet, even a limited one, is variety, or at least as much variety as your child's sensitivities allow. Just keep this mantra in mind: *Diversity is good.*

Cooking for the Food-Sensitive Child

If you like to cook, there are some great recipes around now to suit almost any sensitivity. Using bean, potato, rice, and other non-wheat flours and baking mixes—which are now readily available in health food stores and some grocery stores—you can make almost any baked goodies, including birthday cakes, that are almost indistinguishable from the wheat-based versions. And you can use replacement substitutes where needed for those with egg and milk sensitivities.

Meals take a little more planning than snacks, but because we started so early, Chris never had to deal with any big changes to his diet. I tend more towards careful menu planning than complicated recipe preparation. Dinner typically consists of an entrée like grilled or baked chicken, or perhaps some lean

17

grilled or broiled steaks or a gluten-free meat or turkey loaf, and vegetables like succotash, baked potatoes, and broccoli.

Nothing fancy, but all prepared from scratch to avoid possibly harmful additives. With microwaves as standard appliances in almost every home, cooking fresh or frozen vegetables has never been easier or healthier. And no one really missed bread except my fussy eater, and she soon learned to do without.

A Great Introduction to Healthy Eating

Of course, some parents really rise to the occasion and exercise culinary skills that could put a professional chef to shame. Janet's secret to successful gluten-free living, she will tell you, is to "Bake, bake, bake." "Our rule has been to keep Michael's life as normal as possible. This has meant a tremendous effort on our part, but has worked well. I have baked for every single school party, scouting event, and church event so that there would be gluten-free food for Michael. I always made whole batches so that the other kids were eating the same thing as Michael and he wasn't singled out by having 'special food'."

In Janet's family, as in ours, everyone happily eats gluten free much of the time. "We all eat gluten-free cookies, muffins, pies, cakes," explained Janet. "I make gluten-free trail mix, we buy gluten-free hot dogs, spaghetti sauce, etc. When I make pasta, I make two separate dishes and I make gluten-free bread only for Michael's consumption. Other than that we all eat basically the same things. We are *so* healthy since none of us eat a lot of pre-packaged food. We eat vegetables, meat, poultry, fish, and lots of fruit all prepared to be gluten free."

As Chris grew older, we put bread back on the table, which has cheered my daughter considerably. And Chris doesn't care, especially if he has his own "special" rice flour bread, which I bake for him in my bread machine or buy commercially made.

The point is that, for the most part, these are ordinary meals requiring no extraordinary cooking skills, only attention to ingredients. Convenience is only barely sacrificed, but a lot is gained in the process for everyone.

For a toddler, it's the perfect introduction to healthy eating. And once I learned what snacks were safe and acceptable, I couldn't tell the difference in a playgroup between the kids munching Cheerios™ and Chris munching Corn Pops™ or rice cakes. As a matter of fact, it wasn't unusual for other kids to want some of HIS snacks instead of theirs!

Taking Food Sensitivities to School
If your child is in preschool, you'll have to make sure the teachers are aware of the problem, and you might want to prepare your own list of snacks and foods that are safe for your child. One useful guide to review with your child's caretakers is "Off to School with Food Sensitivities: A Guide for Parents and Teachers" from the Food Allergy Network.[10]

You also need to make sure birthday and other celebrations don't endanger your child with the wrong foods. If you know in advance when parties are planned, you can make up special snacks that are okay for your child, and that all the other children will enjoy, too. (See Chapter 11 for great party fixes!)

Snacks for preschoolers and older children might include:

- Carrot sticks & (safe) dips
- Chips (apple, corn, potato)
- Dates
- Fruit (fresh, dried, canned)
- Popsicles
- Raisins
- Rice crackers with suitable toppings
- Seeds (pumpkin, sunflower)

---

[10] To order this 2-booklet set contact The Food Allergy Network, 10400 Eaton Place, Suite 107, Fairfax, VA 22030-2208, or visit their web site at http://www.foodallergy.org. Contact: Michael Geylin of Kermish-Geylin Public Relations, 212-315-4900, for The Food Allergy Network.

- Juices (100% pure)
- Popcorn

- Trail mix (seeds, nuts, M&Ms™) [11]

> *"When my son started at a new daycare I explained his dietary limitations and that I would be supplying all his food. That evening when I came to pick up my kids, there was Cody with a bright yellow sign stuck on both front and back of his shirt.... Do Not Feed Me! The daycare owner had done this in order not to have a mistake made when all the staff was interacting with Cody. I thought it was a wonderful idea and have used it at gatherings since. The sign I pinned on Cody would say, "Please don't feed me until you check with my Mom and Dad". I used this until he was able to communicate on his own. He was 20 months when diagnosed and is now almost seven."*—Karen

Empowering Your Child

Educating your child early on gives him a sense of responsibility for his own health and diet, and that goes a long way toward keeping him safe and healthy. "My job is to help him learn how to *live* with his condition," says Lindsay. "Sam's diet is different and the sooner he comes to terms with that the better."

Tracey helped put Kevin in charge of his diet right from the start. "Parents should immediately start teaching their child that gluten is bad for them—even if the child is a baby. Kevin at 2 1/2 years old already knows that gluten will hurt him, and he "reads" food labels when we're shopping. It's never too early to start teaching them."

Some children enjoy fixing their own meals and snacks that everyone can enjoy. Let your child control his health by becoming familiar with the foods that are best for him and he'll be less likely to eat the wrong things when he's away from you. Make sure he understands what causes his discomfort when he eats the wrong foods, and that he can explain his situation clearly to others. If he can learn to manage his own dietary environment,

---

[11] It should go without saying—but I'll say it anyway—that any snack mixes you put together should take the sensitivities of other children into consideration. Don't use nuts in your gluten-free mix, for instance, if you think there may be sensitivities to nuts in your child's group.

he's less likely to feel like the victim of an illness beyond his control, or to be treated as one. Remember, the goal is to help your child *eat differently without feeling different.*

Learning to manage Chris' diet taught us not to make food an issue for him. We never used food for bribery or as a reward. And since food never took on emotional associations for him, he was much more matter-of-fact about what he ate. Food is fuel and should be treated as such. His is just high octane, that's all.

In that way, we were able to build caution into him instead of fear. From his perspective, there's plenty to choose from; it's just a matter of choosing the right thing.

Early on, Chris learned to express himself quite clearly about what he could and couldn't eat. He knew cookies were out and his first clear sentence was "No thank you, I'm 'lergic to wheat." Technically, that might not be correct, but it was easy to say and he got his point across. We couldn't be prouder, both because he never felt driven by a desire for cookies and because he showed such self-control and self-possession.

I'm convinced that his mild character has a lot to do with his diet, which is extremely healthy. Not that he isn't as rambunctious as any boy. He talks non-stop, has a stubborn streak, and his hugs can break bones. But he knew self-control at an early age and we can always

> *"You feel so much better if you stay on your diet. You have energy and you feel almost normal."*—Jessica, 16

rely on him to behave himself under the most demanding circumstances. If that doesn't speak for diet, I don't know what does. If Chris's condition has taught me nothing else, it's affirmed for me that we really are what we eat.

21

Karen, too, has worked from the very beginning to teach Cody how to live with his condition. "One time at a family reunion," she recalled, "Cody was at another family's campsite when they were making S'mores (a graham cracker and chocolate bar treat). The mom tried to give Cody a graham cracker. He was just three years old and he had never seen a cracker like this before. He told the lady," No, me sick." He knew enough not to eat it and I give him tons of credit for taking his own diet under control and managing it at such a young age."

Good Diets Make For Good Health
It only stands to reason that eating a good, healthy diet at an early age can facilitate a good quality of life. Everything we've seen has shown us that, especially the changes we saw immediately following the improvement in Chris' diet. His severe stuttering cleared up, he became dry through the night within just a couple of weeks of eliminating wheat from his diet, and even his learning skills seemed to improve.

So in just a few short months, we had learned to adapt to an essentially major dietary change for an American family and, like many others, seen some glowing results in the process. And because we all adapted with a minimum of fuss, our little boy adapted with ease and compliance.

In retrospect, the changes were not all that earth shattering. We had gone from Cheerios™ to Corn Pops™; from cookies and teething toast to rice crackers and pieces of apple, cut up grapes and carrot sticks; from rolls and whole wheat bread with dinner to corn bread if we needed any bread at all.

The hard part seemed done. We were eating natural; now we just had to make it *look* natural!

Summing It All Up

● *Trust your instincts*. Ask questions and learn where to look for answers. *There's no substitute for a well-informed parent.* Look for educational and moral support groups in your area so you can learn from other parents and share ideas.

● *Don't go it alone!* Find a good pediatric gastroenterologist, allergist, dietitian, nutritionist, or physician familiar with food sensitivities who will work closely with you and your child to help manage his or her diet safely.

● *Food sensitivities affect up to 6% of children, possibly as many as 34 million Americans.* Technically, a "food allergy" is an immune response to a food, and a food intolerance, while creating similar symptoms, does not involve the immune system. Whether your child suffers from an allergy or from an intolerance (we'll use the word "sensitivity" to cover the whole spectrum), if you suspect your child is sensitive to a food, explore that suspicion. Ask your health professional about removing the suspect food on a trial basis.

● *Well-meaning physicians can be slow to diagnose food sensitivities* in children because symptoms often mimic those of common childhood problems like colds, flu, stomach virus and reactions to antibiotics. Parental insistence on getting to the true source of a problem is often the only way to get a correct diagnosis.

● The *earlier* food sensitivities are identified, the sooner your child can be comfortable and happy, and begin to grow properly and develop to his or her best potential.

● *Get educated about your child's food sensitivities*. Ask questions in the health food store and explore web sites. Learn to read labels and become familiar with the various forms your child's target food can take.

● *KISS*: Keep it Simple and Safe. The fewer ingredients in the

23

foods you feed your food-sensitive child, the better. Use pure, wholesome, fresh fruits and vegetables as much as possible, in a diet that emphasizes diversity as much as possible.

- *Empower your child* by teaching him early on how to control and manage his own diet. The more confident your child is, the less "different" your child will feel, and the healthier your child will be—for life.

Chapter II
Amber Waves of Grain:
A World of Wheat

My world was awash in wheat when Chris was born. Our growing family went through loaves of bread with gusto, enjoying hot buttered toast for breakfast, sandwiches for lunch, and buttered slices of bread with dinner. Five pound bags of flour were no match for our hungry brood, who loved pancakes, birthday cakes, cupcakes, and muffins. Every holiday our home was deep in the aroma of baked cookies, pies, and breads. We just loved our wheat!

But it just didn't seem to agree with my tender-tummied toddler. No sooner did Chris eat than we had to change a messy diaper. Or, in the early stages of potty training, we had to make a bee-line for the bathroom. The volume of his stool was astounding and seemed far out of proportion to what he was eating—although he had a hefty appetite that rarely seemed satisfied. I couldn't see how he was getting anything out of the food he was eating when it seemed to course through his body so quickly.

But he was never sick, never complained and at every routine doctor visit, he checked out fine. I felt silly asking the doctor about it, but on a couple of occasions brought up my concern. I got vague replies, from suggestions of a virus to simply a delicate stomach. When I queried about the possibility of Crohn's Disease, which my husband has, I was assured that Crohn's doesn't appear until much later in life. But neither our pediatrician nor our family doctor ever suggested a food sensitivity.

I felt like I was worrying needlessly, but I worried nonetheless. Compared with my two other children, Chris' bathroom habits seemed especially unusual. While evidently healthy otherwise, he was very slender, at the bottom of the weight chart, with a pot-belly and that "wasted buttocks" look that I later learned was often associated with celiac disease and other malabsorption problems.

On a hunch, and guided by some medical literature I'd found, I decided to try removing wheat from Chris' diet for a trial period. Within a matter of weeks, his bloating and diarrhea had cleared up. His stools looked normal and were reduced considerably in both frequency and volume.

We were freed from the bathroom at last and Chris, while he hadn't acted ill or complained in any way[12], was delighted as well. We could go out now and do things we couldn't do before because we had to be sure we were near a restroom at all times. Now we could go to parks and to the beach. He began to put on weight, speak more clearly, and he became dry through the night.

Wheat Sensitivity

When taking wheat out of Chris' diet met with such immediate success, I became curious about the mechanisms behind this food sensitivity. I discovered that wheat sensitivities, like other food sensitivities, come in various forms and sizes and are neither unprecedented nor uncommon.

Wheat, like most foods, is composed of a number of different types of proteins[13], which can trigger adverse reactions in sensitive individuals. Wheat proteins are found in the

---

[12] Children with food sensitivities may not complain of any discomfort or feel any pain. I mention this to serve as a warning that lack of pain or discomfort doesn't mean that food sensitivities aren't causing harm or that your child doesn't have a serious medical problem if his body is reacting improperly to certain foods. Check with your child's doctor if you have any concerns.

[13] Oregon State University Extension Service, Cereals Specialist Russ Karow, "A Wheat Quality Primer", April 1998.

endosperm of the wheat kernel, the part of wheat used in making flours and cereals.

The endosperm is mostly starch, with about 8-15% comprised of four different types of proteins: albumins, globulins, gliadins, and glutenins. Albumins and globulins are water soluble, biologically active proteins that help break down starch. Gliadins and glutenins are storage proteins, collectively called "gluten," and most commonly associated with wheat flours.

Gluten is what gives bread dough the spongy elasticity that helps trap air bubbles produced by yeast and other leavening agents that make bread rise. Besides wheat, gluten proteins are also found in other members of the grass family including barley, rye, spelt, and triticale, and occur in products made of these grains, as well.

Things like malt, hydrolyzed vegetable/plant proteins, textured vegetable proteins, soy sauce, grain alcohol, natural flavors, and many of the binders and fillers found in vitamins and medications *may* contain gluten and can trigger a response in sensitive individuals. The only treatment for celiac disease and other wheat sensitivities is a diet free of wheat, barley, and rye and, traditionally, oats, although recent research suggests that *uncontaminated* oats *may* be safe for celiacs.[14]

Generally speaking, when the gluten protein triggers a reaction, an individual is said to have celiac sprue, gluten sensitivity enteropathy, or just simply celiac disease. When the triggering protein cannot be specifically identified, or is attributed to fractions of several proteins, an individual is said to be wheat-

---

[14] Hoffenberg, Ed. M.D.

sensitive. Either way, wheat and its constituent grains cause similar symptoms.[15]

Plop, plop, fizz, fizz

Reactions to allergens can manifest themselves in any of four different ways[16] called, appropriately enough, Type I, Type II, Type III, and Type IV reactions. The types of reactions we're usually talking about when we're discussing food sensitivities are Type I, Immediate Hypersensitivity, IgE mediated responses, and Type IV, Delayed Hypersensitivity, or cell-mediated responses. Type I reactions include things like allergic rhinitis, asthma, food allergies and intolerances, and anaphylactic reactions.

Whether reactions are immediate or take days to occur, however, symptoms are often similar, and frequently gastrointestinal in nature, including abdominal pain, bloating, gas, nausea, vomiting, and diarrhea.

Other symptoms include skin reactions like hives, eczema or dermatitis, mouth ulcers and, in the case of celiac disease, a blistery, itching rash called dermatitis herpetiformis (DH). And symptoms can also be flu-like in nature, including headache, nasal congestion, and rhinitis, general aches and pains, restlessness, and irritability.

With such wide-ranging and general symptoms, it's easy to see why wheat (and other) food sensitivities can be hard to pin down. Diagnostic techniques vary according to suspicions.

---

[15] Taylor, Steve L., Ph.D., University of Nebraska, "Prospects for the Future: Emerging Problems—Food Allergens", presented at Conference on International Food Trade, Beyond 2000: Science-Based Decisions, Harmonization, Equivalence and Mutual Recognition, Melbourne. Australia, October 1999
[16] Merck Manual, 1999

28

Catching the Culprit

In almost all cases, a detailed medical and dietary history is taken and then one or more of several diagnostic methods are used to find the problem. Skin and blood tests are often the first course of action. Then elimination diets and food challenges are next, depending on the results of the more traditional lab work.

Not all food sensitivities show up on skin prick tests or in all blood screenings, though, and celiac disease has the distinction of being one of them. That's why a trial removal of wheat is a helpful test, and in our case, provided the necessary circumstantial evidence to keep wheat away for good. Whether the diagnosis was celiac disease or wheat sensitivity seemed a moot point to us, since the treatment is almost identical: no wheat.

But if your child has been diagnosed as having celiac disease, you need to avoid the additional grains mentioned earlier: barley, rye, spelt, triticale (and possibly oats). And you might be interested in learning that it's not as "rare" a disease as once thought.

Celiac Disease

Celiac disease is an autoimmune disorder, meaning that the body's immune system attacks its own organs and tissues as the "enemy" in addition to intruding organisms like viruses or bacteria. In celiac disease, the immune system reacts to gluten (more specifically, the gluten protein gliadin) by damaging the villi, the little fingerlike projections that line the small intestine and aid in the absorption of nutrients. That can lead to malnutrition and other problems.

Very recent research has found that the human protein "zonulin" plays a role in celiac disease. When working properly, zonulin acts as a "gatekeeper of our body's tissues. " However, researchers at the University of Maryland discovered that celiac patients have increased levels of zonulin, which makes the "gateways" between cells stick open and inadvertently allows the gluten protein to pass through to the immune system where it's attacked by antibodies, leading to the autoimmune disorder.[17]

Celiac disease tends to run in families. That doesn't mean that ancestors or more immediate relatives were necessarily diagnosed with celiac disease, but that they may have had, or do suffer from, associated autoimmune disorders such as diabetes mellitus (insulin dependent)—which both my son's paternal grandfather and maternal great-grandmother had—thyroid disease, Sjogren's syndrome, systemic lupus erythematosus (SLE), or rheumatoid arthritis, to name a few. Often too, those afflicted with Addison's disease and Down syndrome suffer from celiac disease.

Medical literature says that the onset of celiac disease typically occurs around two years of age, after wheat has been introduced into the diet. As a matter of fact, studies comparing rates of celiac disease in various countries have found that countries with high frequency and duration of breastfeeding (six months or more) and commensurately delayed introduction of grains into infant diets seems to significantly reduce the incidence of celiac disease.[18]

But there is no hard and fast rule; celiac disease can begin anytime wheat gluten finally triggers an inflammatory reaction in the small bowel sufficiently large enough to damage large numbers of villi. Once the villi are damaged, there is less

---

[17] The same research found that zonulin may also contribute to the development of other autoimmune disorders like insulin dependent diabetes and multiple sclerosis, Fasano, Alessio, M.D., "Researchers find increased zonulin levels among celiac disease patients," Lancet, April 2000.

[18] Ascher, Henry, M.D., "Quality and Quantity of Grains in the European Diet," 9th International Celiac Symposium, Baltimore, MD, August 2000.

30

intestinal surface area to absorb nutrients, fluids, and electrolytes, which often result in the messy, frequent bowel movements celiacs may experience.

Symptoms can actually vary a lot. In fact, the majority of individuals have *no* symptoms. If there is significant intestinal damage, symptoms can include diarrhea, weakness, and weight loss. If intestinal damage is less significant, nutrient and fluid absorption will be unaffected and symptoms can manifest themselves more obscurely with problems such as anemia-related fatigue. Sometimes the only symptom is short stature, due to insufficient absorption of calcium and other nutrients[19] but others include osteopenic bone disease, tetany (muscle spasms) and neurologic disorders. Sometimes a blistering, burning, itchy rash called dermatitis herpetiformis occurs with celiac disease.

It is unknown at this time whether gluten-sensitive individuals will actually develop the clinical symptoms of celiac disease over time. What is known is that removing gluten from the diet of either clinically active celiac disease patients or those with antibodies present can regenerate the intestinal surface area and resolves the symptoms experienced by most patients.[20]

Early Detection Helps
It's interesting to note that celiac disease is the most common genetic disorder in Europe. (It rarely occurs in those of African, Chinese, or Japanese descent.) One in 250 people are diagnosed with celiac disease in Italy and about one in 300 in Ireland.[21]

---

[19] This is a little known and poorly recognized symptom of celiac disease, despite the fact that there is significant evidence suggesting that up to 20% of children measuring below the 5th percentile in height may suffer from undiagnosed celiac disease. In many of these cases, short stature was the *only* symptom of celiac disease. Hoggan, Ronald, "How Often is Short Stature Predictive of Celiac Disease?" University of Calgary.

[20] Pruessner, Harold T., M.D, "Detecting celiac disease in your patients," American Family Physician, American Academy of Family Physicians, 1998

[21] Read the entire overview in NIH Publication Number 98-4225. Updated March 25, 1999

31

That would make it as common as milk, egg, and peanut sensitivities among children.

It's believed that celiac disease is under-diagnosed in the U.S., especially since the disorder is genetic and many Americans descend from European ethnic groups who are susceptible to the disease. In the spring of 1998, scientists at the Center for Celiac Research at the University of Maryland Medical Center launched a nationwide three-year Serological Screening Study to determine the incidence of celiac disease in the United States.

Just one year into the study, doctors discovered a large ratio of patients studied had celiac antibodies even though they show no symptoms. By August, 2000, the Screening Study had evaluated 10,000 individuals and released preliminary data showing that as many as one in every 120 Americans may have celiac disease. This is much higher than the official one in 4,700 actually diagnosed with the ailment.[22]

The longer celiac disease goes undiagnosed and untreated, the greater the chances of malnutrition and other complications. In Italy, where the disease is common, all children are routinely screened for celiac disease by age six. And when Italians of any age show symptoms, they are tested for celiac disease immediately. The result of such vigilance is that it typically only takes two to three weeks to diagnose celiac disease in Italy—in stark contrast to the average, and maddeningly slow, diagnosis time of almost ten years in the U.S. (NIH Publication Number 98-4225.)

---

[22] For more information or to participate in the study, contact Dr. Alessio Fasano, Professsor of Pediatrics and Medicine, through the University Physicians Consultation and Referral Service, 1-800-373-4111.

Celiac Specific Testing

The most common way to test for celiac disease, when anyone thinks to do it at all, consists of a blood screening followed by endoscopic biopsy. The blood labs look for three specific antibodies called IgA, IgE, and IgG (and something new called tTG, that I'll explain in a minute). Try not to let all the acronyms get to you, and I'll try to explain what they are, courtesy of the Center for Celiac Research (CCR) at the University of Maryland in Baltimore.

- IgA antiendomysial antibodies (AEA) are specific to celiac disease and dermatitis herpetiformis.

- IgE gamma globulin antibodies are produced by cells lining the intestinal wall and respiratory tracts, and often associated with allergic responses like asthma and hayfever.

- IgG is the main immunoglobulin in our blood.

Both IgA and IgG anti-gliadin antibodies (AGA) are detected in celiac patients. IgG anti-gliadin antibodies are more sensitive but are less specific markers for celiac disease than IgA class antibodies.

Typically, if a patient is IgA positive, then there's more than a 90% chance he has celiac disease. Patients who are IgG positive may have problems similar to celiac disease, but not specifically have the disease. Consequently, patients suspected of having celiac disease are usually tested for both IgA and IgG antibodies, which together are 90% accurate in detecting celiac.

To Biopsy or Not to Biopsy

Because we cleared Chris' problems up directly, through diet, our doctor saw no need for a biopsy—given his age and lack of any other symptoms—unless we wanted a specific diagnosis of celiac disease. While new tests are becoming available and increasingly more reliable, a biopsy remains the only way to definitively diagnose the ailment. But in order for a biopsy to be effective, Chris had to go back to his old diet and damage his gut again for accurate results.

There are two sides to this issue: On the one hand, a biopsy would determine categorically if Chris actually and undeniably suffers from celiac disease. It might also pinpoint another problem, if it wasn't celiac disease. On the other hand, since the only treatment for celiac disease is a wheat-free/gluten-free diet, and going on a wheat-free/gluten-free diet had already eliminated his gastrointestinal and other symptoms, it seemed—to us at least—counterproductive to put him back on wheat to prove he was, indeed, sensitive to wheat.

And then there's a third hand. Dr. Kenneth Fine, a gastroenterologist in the process of developing new testing technology, notes, "Although by definition a normal small bowel biopsy rules out celiac sprue, it does not rule out gluten sensitivity. Although asymptomatic people with gluten sensitivity may have normal or near-normal biopsies, so too may people with symptomatic gluten sensitivity. This has been reported in the medical literature (called "Gluten Sensitivity with Minimal Enteropathy" or "Gluten-Sensitive Diarrhea without Celiac Disease")." [23]

Do understand, though, that a biopsy is still considered the only way to actually confirm celiac disease. Some people feel it is worth the temporary discomfort of returning gluten to the diet to confirm celiac disease through a biopsy and rule out other disorders. Biopsy-confirmed patients are preferred in medical

---

[23] Fine, Kenneth, M.D., "Diagnosis of Gluten Sensitivity in the 21st Century: Time for A Change," FinerHealth and Nutrition <www.finerhealth.com> , EnteroLab <www.enterolab.com> , and the Intestinal Health Institute, Dallas, Texas.

research.[24] And, since biopsy is the "gold standard" for celiac diagnosis only biopsied patients are counted in official statistics. However you lean on the issue, I want to emphasize that this is an important decision that you should make under the guidance of a physician, as we did.

New and Improved

But new developments are on the horizon. A few years ago, a new antibody enzyme was discovered in Germany and given the name "tissue transglutaminase"or tTG. This newly discovered antibody is highly sensitive. In clinical trials at the University of Maryland's Center for Celiac Research, it has been nearly 100% correct in diagnosing celiac disease. A new diagnostic test that screens for this antibody, known as the tTG ELISA test, can be conducted within 30 minutes at a participating physician's office. Currently, there are studies underway to see if the Human tTG dot-blot test might eventually replace intestinal biopsy as the "gold standard" for celiac diagnosis.[25]

Other forms of testing also look promising. Dr. Fine believes gluten sensitivity (and other food sensitivities) can be detected earlier and with greater accuracy through stool rather than blood samples.[26] The hope here is that a diagnosis can be made before there is ever any damage to the intestinal villi.

Up and Coming

And one day, there may not even be damage to the villi at all, if Dr. Bob Buchanan's work continues to show progress. A professor at the University of California at Berkeley and a former Chair of the Department of Plant and Microbial Biology at the University, Dr. Buchanan is leading research into the genetic

---

[24] Don Kasarda, Ph.D: Gluten Intolerance Group of North America Conference, Seattle 2000

[25] Center for Celiac Research, University of Maryland

[26] See www.finerhealth.com or www.enterolab.com for more information

use of a small protein located outside the chloroplasts of plants called thioredoxin h.

Thioredoxin h degrades protein and starch reserves in grains. In vitro experiments have shown that it can alleviate food and pollen allergies, enhance digestibility and nutritional qualities of foods and improve the baking quality of poor quality flours. The same technology may also eventually be applied to reducing the allergenic properties of peanuts, soy, and milk. (Thioredoxin also disarms the neurotoxins of snakes, scorpions and bees, but that's another story!)

In an address to the Senate Committee on Agriculture, Nutrition, and Forestry in October 1999, Dr. Buchanan said, "It is our goal that someday food products containing cereals will be formulated with hypoallergenic grain so that persons with cereal allergies can eat a wide range of food products without fear of significant health related injuries or concerns."[27]

But until that scenario becomes a reality, a gluten-free diet is the only treatment.

Embracing the New Diet

Now, we just had to learn how to make Chris' diet a part of our lives, as well as an accepted and normal part of his—forever. Although some early literature suggested he might outgrow his sensitivity to wheat, more contemporary studies confirm that it is a lifetime condition. Only the symptoms *might* disappear in adolescence. The gluten (or other protein) still does its damage,

---

[27] Statement of Bob B. Buchanan, Ph.D., Professor University of California, Berkeley, California Senate Committee on Agriculture, Nutrition, and Forestry, October 6, 1999. "Dr. Bob Buchanan Explains How His Research Using Plant Biotechnology Is Removing Allergens from Existing Foods, "American Society of Plant Physiologists, <http://www.aspp.org/pubaff/tesbuch.htm >

just without as much discomfort, and the chances of incurring more far reaching problems like arthritis, neurological problems, and other ailments due to nutritional deficiencies can be higher.

In fact, there is compelling data to suggest that a gluten-free diet reduces the significantly higher risk of intestinal cancers like lymphoma and adenocarcinoma that are associated with untreated celiac disease.[28] And even more recent research has found that the risks of developing other autoimmune disorders are lessened if celiac disease is identified and treated early.[29] Other problems that can arise from damage to the intestines and malnutrition caused by untreated celiac disease include osteoporosis, short stature, and seizures.

No, everything we read pointed to the fact that Chris had to be wheat-free for life. And others we'll meet here have to be milk-

> "It's better not to have wheat when you're allergic to it, even if you can't have certain things to eat. I don't even like eating wheat now. I feel a whole lot better when I don't eat wheat."
> —Chris, 7

free for life, or avoid peanuts or eggs forever. The change of diet for a food-sensitive child is permanent and unyielding and necessary for good health and a good quality of life.

Where's the Wheat?
If it were just a matter of getting rid of bread and looking for the word "wheat" on labels, managing a wheat-free diet would be— pardon the pun—a piece of cake. As you'll find, though, there's a lot more to wheat than meets eye, or the palate.

---

[28] National Digestive Diseases Information Clearinghouse, National Institutes of Health (NIH) Publication No. 98-4269, April 1998.
[29] Ventura, Alessandro, M.D., "Celiac Disease and Autoimmunity: Which Comes First?" 9th International Celiac Symposium, Baltimore, MD, August 2000.

Wheat is a staple food product in the United States. It's in nearly all baked goods, used as a thickener in sauces, puddings and soups, dusted on candy, and used in colorings and flavorings. It can hide in additives such as mono and digylcerides, in dextrins and hydrolyzed vegetable protein.

If your child is gluten sensitive, you'll also need to avoid bran, couscous, durum, semolina, spelt and kamut, in addition to wheat, barley, and rye.

Now a note about oats here: Most literature recommends avoiding them. More contemporary studies say the biggest problem with oats is the possibility of cross-contamination with wheat due to shared processing facilities.[30] In fact, Dr. Edward Hoffenberg and fellow researchers at Children's Hospital in Denver, CO, found that newly diagnosed celiac children had no adverse effects from eating oats on a short-term basis. But this doesn't mean they're safe for long-term consumption. (Their findings will be published in the Journal of Pediatrics). So, while moving up on the acceptance scale, oats are still not recommended in the gluten-free diet.

Wheat: It's not the only thing to eat
Of course knowing where the wheat is and learning to get along without it are two different things. We're creatures of habit and it's largely habit that drives our diet and the diet we model for our children. We eat out of habit and we eat the same things out of habit, and sweet things made out of wheat top the list.

---

[30] In the spring of 2000, Finish researchers concluded preliminary studies that found that people with celiac disease who eat oats show no adverse auto-antibody or intraepithelial lymphocyte level effects. According to the researchers, these results" strengthen the view that adult patients with celiac disease can consume moderate amounts of oats without adverse immunological effects," however, "more clinical studies are needed to ensure the safety of oats when consumed permanently in a celiac diet as well as to determine the effect of larger amounts of oats." Janatuinena, E.K. et al., "Lack of cellular and humoral immunologial responses to oats in adults with coeliac disease, Gut 2000, 46: 327-331. March 10, 2000.

Living wheat free requires a major change of attitude. In and of itself, living without wheat is not all that difficult. But in and of itself, changing our attitude, making the all-important paradigm shift from bread being the staff of life to the stuff of discomfort and illness—*that* can be difficult.

But once you take that leap of logic, once you decide your child's health is more important than habit, once you start looking at diet from the outside, a whole new world will open up for your child and for your whole family. Wheat, you'll discover, isn't the only thing to eat.

Fresh vegetables and fruits, safe grains like rice and corn, lean meats and vegetables all make great meals without a grain of wheat in them. There are whole lines of wheat and gluten-free products available now, and wheat and gluten-free baking

> *"I'd just like people to know that going by the diet has a lot better results than having convenience in eating. You feel a lot better. Ever since I was 9, I have had this idea for a restaurant called the 'Silly Yak' for celiacs. Celiacs would contribute recipes and cooking techniques and only celiacs could be chefs. The animal (like the Taco Bell™ dog or Colonel Sanders™ or Ronald McDonald™) would be a blue yak. There would be every gluten-free recipe under the sun. "*—Nicole, 12

mixes that enable you to make convincingly wheat-like treats without the commensurate problems. There are enough wheat-free recipes in this book alone to keep you and your children happy and healthy for a long time to come!

It's All in the Attitude
It's up to you to model a good attitude for your wheat-sensitive child. Without you showing the way—or with you apologizing or feeling sorry for your child because of his "problem"—your child will not be able to make the necessary attitude adjustments himself, especially if he's older than a toddler.

When we discovered Chris' problem, we never even blinked. Well, maybe I blinked a little, but I didn't let him see me! We just went right on like nothing had happened. Whole wheat breads disappeared from the table and were replaced with corn bread. Chicken was breaded in potato chips or corn croutons instead of bread crumbs. Instead of toast for breakfast with wheat-based cereals, we found ourselves eating pancakes—rice flour pancakes—or scrambled eggs. Instead of cookies for a snack, we ate trail mixes, Jello®, or fruit cups.

Basically, we just didn't make a big deal out of it. And neither did Chris. He ate what was on the table and rarely noticed that what was on the table didn't include wheat. Eating out took a little practice (we'll cover that in detail later), but we learned how to order grilled or broiled meats and poultry, burgers without buns, and baked potatoes instead of fries to lessen the chance of wheat-based seasonings.

We brought our own special treats to parties and outings. Corn chips and safe potato chips, homemade dips, safe party mixes and wheat-free brownies and fudge. And Chris learned quickly and easily when to say, "No, I can't eat that," and when to say, "Thanks!"

Once we made that paradigm shift, once we got our footing and adjusted our attitudes, life without wheat was, indeed, a piece of cake!

Summing it All Up

- *Wheat sensitivities result from an inability to digest any or all of the proteins in the endosperm of wheat.* When gluten triggers a reaction, celiac disease results. When the triggering protein cannot be specifically identified, or is attributed to fractions of several proteins, the diagnosis is wheat-sensitivity. Either way, wheat and its constituent grains cause similar symptoms. These include:
  - Chronic diarrhea, often gassy and explosive, with a characteristic greenish color—and difficult to flush away. This is caused by damage to the villi—the fingerlike protrusions in the intestines that aid in absorption of nutrients—and results in malnutrition and other problems.
  - Fussiness and irritability
  - A consequent failure to thrive
  - ADHD-like symptoms and learning disabilities may also accompany celiac disease in children.

- *Celiac disease is an autoimmune disorder that requires different diagnostic tests. Although once considered "rare," it may affect more people than current U.S. statistics show, possibly as many as 1 in 120 Americans.*

- *Although some early literature suggested that celiac disease might be outgrown, more contemporary studies confirm that it is a lifetime condition.*

- *There's more to wheat than meets the eye or the palate. All forms of wheat must be avoided, including barley, rye, spelt, triticale, kamut, and possibly oats—which are gluten-free, but have not received official endorsement for celiacs because of possible contamination. Wheat can be found in:*
  - Nearly all baked goods,
  - Thickeners in sauces, puddings, and soups,
  - Dusting on candy,
  - Some flavorings (beware of "natural flavors") and colorings (although caramel coloring is gluten free)
  - Additives such as mono and digylcerides, dextrins, and hydrolyzed vegetable/plant protein.

41

- *Once you start looking at diet from the outside, a whole new world will open up for your child and for your whole family. Wheat, you'll discover, isn't the only thing to eat. You can still enjoy:*
- Fresh vegetables and fruits,
- Safe grains like rice and corn,
- Lean meats and vegetables
- Wheat-free commercial products
- Wheat-free baking mixes and recipes

- *It's up to you to model a good attitude for your wheat sensitive child. With practice, life without wheat can be a piece of cake!*

Chapter III
"Got Water?"
Going Dairy Free in the Land of Milk and Honey

If anything is more of a staple in American diets than wheat, it would have to be cow's milk. While people often seem to accept that adults may not be able to tolerate milk, explaining that your baby or toddler can't have milk is a whole 'nuther thing.

With babies and toddlers, going milk-free seems a special affront to everything childhood represents. Babies and milk are just a given, as far as most people are concerned. Babies naturally evoke Norman Rockwell images of cows and barns and of that warm, supposedly life-giving liquid swirling in pails. A glass of milk with cookies after school, little cubes of cheese for fat toddler fingers, ice cream with birthday cake; for most people it's hard to find more comforting visions than these. For children with lactose or cow milk allergy, however, they amount to torture (not to mention that cake and cookies for those who are gluten intolerant, too!)

Adverse Reactions to Milk
According to the National Institutes of Health, as many as 30 to 50 million Americans are lactose intolerant. Figures are higher for those of African or Asian descent, ranging from as much as 75% of African Americans suffering from lactose intolerance to 90% of Asian Americans (NIH publication No. 98-275).

The Allergy Society of South Africa, a country where the majority of citizens are sensitive to milk, suggests cow milk allergy is so common "perhaps because it is usually the first foreign protein (substance) encountered by infants.

"Cow milk allergy (CMA) affects about 2 to 7.5% of infants. Unfortunately, some CMA patients may develop an allergy to

43

other food proteins (e.g. egg, soy, peanut) and some may develop an allergy to one or more inhalant allergens (e.g. grass pollens, house dust mite, cat) before puberty. There is also a higher risk of developing other allergic diseases such as asthma or eczema."[31]

Milk contains a number of allergens, but the two main culprits are whey and casein, and problems can develop with either or both. Technically, casein is the "curd" that forms when milk sours, and whey is what is left after the curd is removed. While both can give Little Miss Muffet a fright, the whey, which comprises 20% of the milk content, causes the most clinical problems. Whey consists mostly of a couple of things called alpha-lactalbumin and beta-lactaglobulin, which are most likely to produce the famous Immunoglobulin E (IgE), the antibodies, which show up in allergic individuals.[32]

Lactose Intolerance

The most common adverse reaction to cow's milk is lactose intolerance. Lactose intolerance is caused by a shortage of the enzyme "lactase" which is usually produced by the small intestine. Lactase is responsible for breaking down lactose (milk sugar) so the blood can absorb it. Lactase deficiency prevents digestion of lactose, which leads to discomforts like nausea, bloating, gas, cramps, and diarrhea. Symptoms can occur anywhere from a half-hour to two hours after eating milk products. The severity of symptoms varies by individual sensitivity.

While lactose intolerance rarely causes more than discomfort, that discomfort can be quite severe, and that's reason enough to reduce or eliminate milk intake. In infants and young children, the greater

---

[31] Dr M. Groenewald: Allergy Society of South Africa.
[32] Ibid.

44

health issue is dehydration from chronic diarrhea caused by lactose intolerance. And lactose intolerance requires care to get enough calcium and other important nutrients.[33] Pediatricians suspecting lactose intolerance often recommend a soy formula. But if the problems don't abate, check the label for casein, which indicates the presence of cow's milk and may also create problems.

Allergy to Casein or Whey

Allergic reactions to casein and/or whey protein are caused by an immunological sensitivity to milk *protein*—rather than the sugar. A reaction to casein or whey can cause breathing problems, hives and rashes, abdominal pain, and possibly serious weight loss. While there are at least 30 types of potentially allergy-causing proteins in milk, casein is the most prevalent. The proteins lactalbumin and lactoglobulin, which comprise the whey proteins, are also known to cause problems.

Because whey proteins are changed by high heat, those sensitive to whey can sometimes tolerate evaporated, boiled, or sterilized milk and milk powder. That other 80% of milk, the casein, is, unfortunately for sensitive folks, heat stable. It's also the most common allergen in cheese, which seems to be particularly craved by those who can't have it. The harder the cheese, the more casein it contains.

And because milk proteins are not altered sufficiently when milk is converted to other dairy products like cheese or yogurt, the only way to avoid reactions is to avoid milk in all its forms.

Interestingly, too, the molecular structure of casein is similar to that of gluten, and those with celiac disease may also suffer from casein intolerance.

---

[33] NIH Publication No. 98-2751

45

Can It Be Outgrown?

Studies show that lactose intolerance often diminishes with age. As for cow milk allergy, allergist Dr. John M. James, a member of the Food Allergy Network (FAN) board, says, "… 80% of children with cow milk allergy can become tolerant to this protein by their third birthday."[34]

Since the literature here, as in other food sensitivities, varies considerably, I'll repeat our dietary management mantra: If your child demonstrates a sensitivity to milk, in addition to removing milk from his or her diet, *it is very important to have the guidance of a good health care practitioner, allergist, nutritionist, dietitian, or pediatric gastroenterologist*. New discoveries about food sensitivities are always being made, and new treatments pioneered. Always keep a good health care professional— especially one with a good understanding of food sensitivities— in your side pocket!

When Milk's Not Good For You

Now, for us, milk wasn't much of an issue because of the overriding concerns of the wheat problem. Chris seemed to have a natural distaste for milk that rather surprised me, but came in handy. I had noticed, after we had cleared up the gluten-induced problems, that he had mild relapses if he had any milk products. We took milk out of his diet along with the wheat and he was fine. He got his calcium and other nutrients from calcium fortified orange juice and from his wheat-free vitamin and mineral supplements.

---

[34] Personal communication with Dr. James. Also, the <u>Allergy Society of South Africa</u> reminds us that CMA may be acquired later in life.

46

But for others, milk may create other issues. Although this work is very controversial, in cases of autism and attention deficit hyperactivity disorder (ADHD), milk *may* actually exacerbate the problem.

Casein and Autism

One of the most intriguing and controversial views about casein concerns its role and that of gluten in autism.[35] Autism is a neurological disorder that usually becomes evident in children between the ages of one and three. Autism affects learning abilities and creates problems in verbal and non-verbal communication as well as in social interaction for afflicted children.

The disorder, which is estimated to occur in as many as one in 500 children (Centers for Disease Control and Prevention, 1997) affects boys four times as often as girls across a non-discriminating range of racial, ethnic, and social backgrounds. Associated behaviors include aggression, self-injury, repetitive body movements such as hand-flapping, and other unusual behaviors.

Although autism is considered one of the most common developmental disorders in the U.S., relatively little is known about its causes. Traditional treatments are not always effective.

Dr. Lisa Lewis, whose son is autistic, was disappointed in his progress with traditional treatments and began exploring connections between autism and diet in an effort to improve her son's progress. Lewis drew on research by the Autism Research Unit of the University of Sunderland in Great Britain which found that about 50% of people with autism have elevated levels of substances similar to opoid peptides (an endorphin-like substance).

---

[35] For more information see Autism Society of America (Associations in Appendix).

47

Casein breaks down in the stomach into a peptide known as casomorphine that has comparable properties. Researchers noted similar effects from wheat gluten and the gluten of other related grains, largely oats, barley, and rye.

Intrigued, Lewis removed both casein and gluten from her son's diet, and wrote a book about her remarkable findings (*Special Diets for Special Kids*, Future Horizons, Inc., 1998). A casein and gluten-free diet, in addition to considerable therapy, improved her son's aggressive behavior and learning abilities in a way that therapy alone seemed unable to achieve.[36]

More recently, author Karyn Seroussi made similarly striking advances with her own autistic son using a casein and gluten-free diet. In her book, *Unraveling the Mystery of Autism and Pervasive Developmental Disorder* (Simon and Schuster, 2000), Seroussi chronicles her son's plunge into autism at the age of 15 months, after a childhood vaccination, which she believes triggered his developmental problems (however, the role of vaccinations in autism is debated) and then back to normal health and development through dietary intervention. Now four, her son is no longer classified as autistic.

Today, Seroussi and Lewis run the Autism Network for Dietary Intervention (ANDI)[37], advocating a gluten and casein free (GFCF) diet for autistic children. Their goal is to help support families who are trying to implement the GFCF diet for autistic and other developmentally disabled children—and to encourage further research into dietary intervention.

---

[36] Lewis, Lisa S., Ph.D., "An Experimental Intervention For Autism: Understanding and Implementing a Gluten & Casein Free Diet," (c) 1994, 1997. <http://members.aol.com/lisas156/gfpak.htm>. Also see <ww.GFCFdiet.com>

[37] See resource section for contact information.

48

Diet and ADHD

A similar (and just as controversial) biology is thought to be at work with ADHD, a learning and behavioral problem that affects an evidently growing number of children each year. Although the complete mechanisms behind how peptides and other molecules affect ADHD is still not completely understood, there is increasing evidence that diet *may* play a role.

While the actual incidence of casein intolerance or celiac disease in ADHD cases may only constitute a small percentage of all cases, Ronald Hoggan, long time researcher and regional director for the Canadian Celiac Association, found, " There is rather a lot of evidence to suggest that extensive exploration of the exorphin hypothesis [opoid peptides] may bring some dramatic changes to that perception."[38]

The idea is certainly getting more attention, but it has yet to be supported by rigorous research. In a study just underway in the spring of 2000 by Dr. Joseph Bellanti, in cooperation with the Georgetown University Medical Center and the University of California at San Francisco, researchers are restricting wheat, dairy, sugar, artificial colors and flavorings from the diets of forty children to examine the impact of dietary restrictions and nutritional supplements on the behavior of children diagnosed with ADHD.

And Dr. Benjamin Feingold, a pediatric allergist from California, has long proposed that salicylates, artificial colors, and artificial flavors, in addition to gluten and casein, can cause hyperactivity and other learning disabilities in children.

---

[38] Hoggan, Ronald, "Application of the Exorphin Hypothesis to Attention Deficit Hyperactivity Disorder: A Theoretical Framework," Dis. University Of Calgary, April 1998.

Miri and Milk

When Miri was born, Linda couldn't have been prouder. A charming, loquacious, inquisitive baby and toddler, Linda and her family suspected nothing more than an "active" child as they watched their daughter grow and blossom.

"Sure, she was not an easy baby, not one who was content to sit for hours and play with her toes," Linda recalled. "She shouted a lot whenever she wanted a new view of the world, and we generally obliged and gave it to her, or a new toy. She had an insatiable curiosity. She was also very outgoing and friendly. She walked quite early, at eight months, before she even crawled..."

But all that energy and boundless enthusiasm didn't translate well into her school years. There were, said Linda, a lot of tears. "They were the hallmark of her kindergarten year. Her teacher, uncharitably, accused Miri of using crying as a manipulative technique designed to get others to do her work for her; she also blamed us for letting her get away with it at home—as much as accusing us of spoiling Miri—but neither of these was true. Miri's tears never got her out of anything, and they weren't a conscious design on her part but rather a clear expression of her extreme frustration at her inability to do as well as she felt she ought to at whatever task."

The following year, a more perceptive teacher pointed out that Miri was having trouble focusing on the tasks at hand. She would spend her time swinging between desks, not listening to instructions, and forgetting to bring class work home. At home, she fared no better, frequently reduced to tears of frustration over her homework.

"The problem was not simply school work. Somewhere between the toddler years and the present, my sweet little baby had gone from a happy-go-lucky child into an often miserable and whiny one. Miri's emotions ran in extremes, buoyant highs, and gruesome lows, with those valleys being so deep that her misery was contagious to all of us around her.

"Despite our best efforts to be positive parents, we spent an awful lot of time with our mouths filled with stupid platitudes of the 'Don't cry over spilled milk' variety, at a loss after all the modern parenting books helped us not at all."

Linda began to explore other options and discovered that Miri was lactose intolerant. Although lactase pills helped the stomach aches she had begun to complain about when she was three, Miri's more immediate problems prevailed. Linda's second child, Ted, was diagnosed with celiac disease, and the family decided to see if that, too,

> *"Being on a milk free diet is VERY hard because you can't have cake* and other stuff. Because if I have milk my stomach starts to hurt and I get mad at small things. Some people say it's weird. Some people say it's CRAZY. But I don't. I mostly get really upset when my mom or brother eats cheese or some sort of cake."*—Miri, 7
> *See Chapter 11 for milk-free cake.

might be Miri's problem. The blood lab came up negative.

Then a chance conversation with a medical transcriber led the family to try removing milk completely from Miri's diet. The change, said Linda, was spectacular.

"The very next day, she was a new kid. It used to be that when it was my night to work in our bookstore, and Dave came with the kids to pick me up, I would start dreading their arrival. When the van pulled up, I could feel myself shrink down, wanting to hide, and listening for the telltale moans and shouts and cries of anger to come from outside the door. Invariably, one or the other or both would be upset. But within 24 hours after we took Miri off of milk, that pretty much stopped happening. Miri started getting along with her brother. She started listening to Dave when he explained math, and clicking to it. She woke up

51

cheerfully, and went to bed cheerfully. Little problems stopped causing major explosions. My sweet baby was back, in a rather grown-up little girl's form, but I could see my cheerful, inquisitive Miri back in blossom again."

"Maybe it's that the discomfort from the lactose intolerance was never entirely relieved by those lactase tablets we gave her. Little kids don't really know what they're supposed to feel like from one moment to the next, I know; so perhaps Miri could not 'put her finger on' whatever was bothering her. I think it's more likely, though, that the lactose intolerance was her body's way of saying that milk just wasn't good for my little girl, that she should stop taking it. I suspect it was interfering with her brain's operation, and I am very glad we tried taking her off of milk." [39]

Linda admits there might be other factors involved in Miri's impressive recovery, but feels removing milk helped significantly. The point is removing milk was worth a try, and in this case proved quite effective.

The Murrays and Milk

For Katherine Murray, her son's adverse reaction to milk proved almost deadly. Her story illustrates, as well, the difficulties encountered in ferreting out the true culprits in food sensitivities

"My older son's first year was a difficult and often unhappy time. From the moment he came home he cried night and day, and was initially diagnosed with colic. He spit up often, and began to scare us with brief bouts of what appeared to be choking. At one month, he stopped breathing in my mother's arms. By the time I picked him up and stimulated him, he recovered his breath."

---

[39] See Linda's website: "ADHD and Living Milk-Free" http://nowheat.com/text/nomilk/)

52

Her son was later admitted to a children's hospital where he was diagnosed with Gastroesophageal Reflux Disease (GERD) and given appropriate medication for the diagnosis. After seven months of adjusting and changing medications, his reflux had eased, but he was still obviously distressed and still suffering from diarrhea. On the advice of a specialist, the family changed their baby's formula to Pregestimil™, a "non-dairy, non-egg, non-soy, casein hydrolysate or predigested formula" (and, adds Katherine, "very expensive") that finally seemed to ease his pain.

The family's reprieve—and the baby's—was only temporary, however. In an effort to find out why Katherine's son continued to suffer pain and bouts of diarrhea, specialists ordered a test called an EGD[40], which would show any internal damage that might have resulted from continued exposure to stomach acid, in the event his reflux was still an issue. Her little boy had to be placed under anesthesia for the test—a frightening prospect for both parents and infants—and biopsies as well as pictures were taken of his esophagus, stomach, and small intestine.

Everything seemed normal. It was several months later that Katherine learned what the problem was. The "dairy-free" Pregestimil® contained 'casein'—a milk protein. "This uncomfortable test could have been avoided if we had known casein was a dairy product," said Katherine. "It is unfortunate that the specialists were also unaware of this unwelcome ingredient." [41]

> *"Being lactose intolerant is nothing you get to choose to be or not to be. It is something that less fortunate people obtain sometime in their life."*
> —Joshua, 12

---

[40] EGD stands for "Esophagogastroduodenoscopy"—basically an upper gastrointestinal endoscopy that visually inspects the gastrointestinal tract by means of a flexible tube and small camera while the patient is lightly sedated.

[41] Read a full discussion of the Murray's experiences on their website, "Children with Milk. Egg and Other Food Allergies" http://users.aol.com/katherinez/kath2.htm#from you

Milk, the Great Masquerader

As with celiac disease, adverse reactions to cow's milk necessitate that parents (and eventually children) become facile label readers. Like the famous actor Lon Chaney, casein has a thousand faces.

"The many hidden sources of milk in processed foods were a real challenge," remembered Edith. "It and its derivatives are everywhere! We learned to read labels compulsively and make most of our foods ourselves. We had to give up most convenience foods."

> "Another thing that I don't like is that it is more difficult to wake up the morning after I have a lot of milk and sometimes I can be late to school and have stomach pains just because of one milkshake or something similar to that."—Jane, 16

Milk masquerades as casein, most often in sodium caseinate; the infamous "milk solids" (curds); whey; lactose (frequently as sodium lactylate); lactalbumin, among others. Be suspicious of anything prefixed "lac." And, beware of all the places milk can crop up, from obvious things like baby formulas to less obvious foods like canned tuna, which may contain hydrolyzed caseinate.

"The general public does not believe in food allergy," says Barbara. "They do not understand that "just a little" can be quite harmful. They think a child with wheat sensitivities just can't eat wheat. It does not dawn on them that wheat is in cookies, cakes, processed chips (Pringles™), crackers, gravies, lunchmeat, etc. They cannot believe you must read every label. And surely they do not comprehend that whey, butter, sodium caseinate, and such are all the same as milk."

Is It a Cold or Milk Allergy?

Almost everyone with a food-sensitive child has to deal with well-meaning folks' insistence that nothing is wrong, despite our strongest convictions to the contrary.

"The pediatrician that I asked told me that I was worrying about toilet training prematurely, since many 3-1/2 year olds are not yet trained," recalled Edith. "But I still knew that something was wrong."

Edith finally saw improvements when she took milk

> *"I found out I was lactose intolerant sometime around the age of five. I was too young to fully understand why my mom was stopping me from eating things like milk, cheese, ice cream, chocolate, etc. As I grew older I became more crafty and sly and would often sneak a bite of that delicious looking fudge. My parents would never find out, but my reactions would remind me after my treat...and my mom would say the classic quote that is still active today, "Joshua, have you had any milk today?"*
> —Joshua, 12

out of her lactose-intolerant daughter's diet. "My daughter had initiated her own toilet training at age 18 months, yet had not had any success for two years. I took her off milk and all derivatives, and within three weeks we saw improvement; it took several more months for all the effects of milk in her diet to fade. The incontinence was the main thing to go (thankfully) but we also noticed an improvement in her sleeping habits and her mood. She was easier to wake up in the morning and less grouchy and difficult in preschool."

Barbara had a similar experience when her original doctor treated her son for pervasive colds and finally pneumonia. A change in doctors brought a change in diagnosis. The new doctor suggested her son had a cow milk allergy, which turned out to be the case.

It's sometimes only through almost superhuman efforts of will that parents of children with food sensitivities finally discover the true problem. They have to run a gauntlet of usually well meaning reassurances that their children have colds or ear infections or "regular" upset stomachs or viruses. Anything, it sometimes seems, but a suggestion that maybe, just maybe, their child can't have milk, or wheat, or peanuts, or eggs. And this is more than unfortunate. It can cause real health problems if children are forced to continue ingesting the foods their bodies are unable to tolerate.

The Dobson-Keeffe's Story

When Rhiannon was born, the Dobson-Keeffe family was delighted with their new baby girl. A charming infant, she thrived until the family tried giving her a bottle of formula when she was nine weeks old. Within thirty minutes, she began projectile vomiting, wheezing and a blotchy red rash covered her body. Several friends of the family had children with gastrointestinal upsets at the time, though, and they didn't make the connection right away.

"We tried her again a week later, choosing a night that was going to be free. Within an hour we had her in emergency in the local hospital. The reactions had been the same as before but her breathing had become very labored and she was constantly choking and gagging on mucus," recalled Rhiannon's father, Nigel, on the website he has devoted to supporting others with similar problems. [42]

The baby was given an antihistamine shot at the hospital and seemed better within half an hour. Doctors there told the family Rhiannon had cow milk allergy and directed them to a local dietitian, where they got mixed results. "They didn't have much information for us and only one old product list for milk-free foods," says Dobson-Keeffe.

---

[42] All references and quotes from the Dobson-Keeffe's are used by permission. Their website is "Milk Allergy and Lactose Intolerance", <http://adelaide.net.au/~ndk/no_milk.htm>

From that outdated list, the Dobson-Keeffe's embarked on the traditional learning journey nearly all parents of children with food sensitivities must take (if they don't have a handy book like this one). Without existing information and good medical and dietary advice to draw from, the parents began educating themselves quite literally from the ground up.

"Eventually we worked out which foods had milk in them and which didn't. We also learned the other names milk products went by. We had a few run-in's with people with no idea, "Oh, there's not much milk in....", "Oh, she can't have milk, can she eat cheese?" All those yummy-looking custards and desserts for babies? Rhiannon never had a single dessert apart from fruit!

"At sixteen weeks we took her back to hospital for a test with a soy-based formula. She was fine. Our next learning task was parties, especially when she could crawl and walk. The only option we ever found was to watch her with eagle eyes. Even if grandma, auntie whoever, or close friends were holding her. It simply wasn't worth the risk."

Rhiannon, now eight, has since learned the ropes of managing her own diet, and the Dobson-Keeffe's report that she's healthy and growing well. If she indulges in milk in any form, they and Rhiannon know immediately. So it doesn't happen very often!

Empowerment is the Key
As always, after the ordeal of identifying the problem, families have to learn how to live with it. Because of milk's prevalence in so many things, from foods to medicines, it takes a little culinary dexterity to negotiate the highways and byways of lactose intolerance or cow milk allergy. Like anything else, though, once you know how, it becomes routine and ordinary. And once again, empowering your children to deal with their food sensitivities is the key to successfully dealing with the

problem. "Teach the child how to read labels," says Barbara. "Before my son could read, someone might ask, 'Matt, can you have these?' showing him the box. He could point to the ingredient label for them to read, subtly reminding them that they (the adult) must make that determination."

Now is as a good a time as any to let your food-sensitive child learn his or her way around the kitchen, too. "This will be a lifetime project for some of them," Barbara reminds us. "They can learn it's fun to cook, and how to make substitutions. They will learn the food groups well enough to eat at restaurants with some good basic reasoning about what they can and cannot order. My son knows

> "The bad thing...is that once you eat the smallest bite of a dairy product you crave it for several days. The food that I respond the worst to has to be cheese. If I eat a pizza (which is often the most tempting food for a child ...) just six hours after I eat my stomach begins to feel upset."
> —Joshua, 12

macaroni and cheese is out of the question, but a hamburger [without the bun] is usually a pretty safe bet."

Learn the Ropes

As far as shopping goes, a few tips can save you time. "If you find the words "parve" or "pareve" on the label, the food is free of all animal and dairy products.[43] This can save you some reading. The words are from Jewish dietary law—they are not allowed to mix milk foods and meat foods, so they must know which foods are neutral", notes Edith.

---

[43] *Typically* (there can be exceptions, as experts remind us) if the product is dairy, it will frequently have a D or the word Dairy next to the kashrut (the K in the circle or a K in a star symbol). If it is pareve (made without milk, meat, or their derivatives) the word Pareve (or Parev) may appear near the symbol. Milchig, another dietary law term, also means made of, or derived from, milk or dairy products. Passover is a great time for the wheat-sensitive to stock up, too, for anything marked "Kosher for Passover"—except matzo in any form—is virtually guaranteed "chametz" or free of wheat, rye, barley, oats, or spelt. Read the labels to be sure.

Shop around, too, says Barbara. "Health food stores and groceries have come a long way. There are so many items available in the past few years that were not common before. [You have to] shop with an open mind. One stop is not going to get it, and that is okay. The prices? Compare them; ask for case prices on things you use a lot. I cook mostly from scratch (no boxed or frozen meals). It is much less expensive, even though the individual ingredients cost more than the standard shelf stock sometimes."

> *"The best advice I can give is this: if you are sensitive to milk it's not worth sneaking that glass of milk, piece of fudge, bowl of cereal, or any other dairy snack."*
> —Joshua, 12

And stand your ground with your children, says Edith. "If the kids whine about not having certain foods, don't argue or explain. They know the whys and wherefores already. Just say, 'Yes, I wish you could have it,

> *"Now that I'm much older my allergy doesn't affect me that much, but if I do drink or eat something with an excess of milk I feel that it's harder for me to wake up and go to school. I sometimes feel like I'm bloated or have gastric problems that are very uncomfortable. It's really my decision to drink/eat milk products and I suffer the consequences on my own."*—Jane, 16

too.' This lets them know you're not depriving them just to be mean or controlling, you're simply dealing with an unpleasant reality."

Both eating out and cooking in will take some planning, but as with anything, practice makes perfect—and so does perspective. "We now eat foods of many more ethnic varieties than I suppose we would otherwise," says Barbara. "Many countries do not have a certain food in their recipes because it is not readily available or something. When you find the right combinations, the flavorful things you can make are endless."

Summing it All Up

- *Adverse reactions to cow milk are common.* According to the National Institutes of Health, as many as 30 to 50 million Americans are lactose intolerant. Figures are higher for those of African (75%) or Asian descent (90%). Furthermore, up to 2.5% of infants develop an allergic reaction to cow milk.

- *Adverse reactions to cow milk are most often manifested in either lactose intolerance—an inability to digest the sugars in milk, or cow milk allergy—an adverse immunologic reaction to milk protein.* Both cause gastrointestinal distress such as diarrhea, nausea, bloating, and vomiting. Sometimes other reactions occur such as hives, rashes, and eczema; cold-like symptoms; general fussiness; chronic ear infections; and anaphylaxis, a severe allergic reaction.

- *The two main allergens in cow milk are "casein," (the curd that forms when milk sours), and " whey," (what is left after the curd is removed) and they appear in many forms in many different kinds of foods, from baby formulas to canned tuna.* They most commonly appear as:
  - Casein, as in sodium caseinate or hydrolyzed caseinate
  - "Milk solids" (curds) or whey
  - Lactose (frequently as sodium lactylate)
  - Lactalbumin and galactose
  - Bovine serum albumin

- *Keep your child's diet varied* within the parameters allowed, and there will be less chance of your child developing additional food sensitivities.

- *Empower your child early* to control his or her own diet

60

Chapter IV
"Aw, Nuts, There's More."
Sensitivities to Peanut, Egg, Corn, Soy, ...

As time went on, I learned more about Chris' new diet and became more adept at dealing with it. I began to discover a lot of things about food in general that I never knew. Several people—from doctors to health food storeowners—cautioned me on several different occasions not to become too reliant on any one alternative food in Chris' diet.

He loved rice crackers, but their tendency to be quickly and easily digested coupled with frequently ingesting them could actually lead to a rice sensitivity, I was told. *That* would certainly put the kibosh on his new dietary lifestyle—and in my choices in providing it to him. When I started to rely more on corn, I was cautioned again that a sensitivity could develop to corn if it, too, was overused.

This definitely required a different mindset from the traditional American dietary habit of grabbing whatever was convenient to feed a child—or oneself. As I spoke to more families and read more medical literature, it began to occur to me that we might be our own worst enemies when it comes to food sensitivities. Our predisposition to eat quickly and conveniently—and to start our children eating the same way in infancy—may lead to the high rate of sensitivities not only to wheat and milk, but also to peanuts, eggs, corn, soy, and, even rice.

And some of these sensitivities can be downright deadly.

Peanuts
Peanuts have the unsavory distinction of causing more severe symptoms than do allergies to other foods, as well as causing

61

higher rates of symptoms with minimal contact.[44] Random surveys have shown a large number of people are allergic to peanuts. While skin prick tests and peanut-specific IgE (that ol' immunoglobulin E) antibody level blood tests (also known as the RAST—radio-allergo-sorbent test) aid in the diagnosis of peanut allergy, they cannot predict the severity of one's reaction to peanuts.

The Kinsley's Story

The Kinsley family found out just how unpredictable peanut sensitivity can be when they gave their year-old son a piece of cracker with peanut butter on it.

"There was no family history of peanut or other food sensitivities, so at about 14 months of age, we tried giving him a little peanut butter on a soda cracker," recalled his father, Steve. "Within a few minutes he began crying severely and rubbing his eyes a lot. After a few more minutes, we saw a bit of swelling around his eyes, but because it was later in the evening, we weren't sure if he was having a reaction or if he was simply over-tired. His crying persisted for about three hours non-stop, much like what had happened when he had croup and had difficulty breathing. In this incident, he ate about half of the cracker (which had a <u>very</u> thin layer of peanut butter)."

The Kinsleys were suspicious but not convinced of anything specific. So they waited a while before trying again.

"We waited for another three to four months and decided to try the same snack (a little peanut butter on a cracker) when we were sure he wasn't over-tired. This time he hardly ate any of the cracker and we did not see a reaction start until about 20 to

---

[44] Weisnagel, John, M.D., "Peanut allergy: where do we stand?, " October 1999, <http://www.allerg.qc.ca/peanutallergy.htm#prev>

30 minutes later. However, when the reaction started, it was much more pronounced than the previous time, with swelling visible not only around the eyes, but also on the face, hands and wrists (blotchy flushing on face as well). Severe crying once again resulted, lasting again for more than three hours non-stop. We interpreted this once again as difficulty breathing."

At their son's regular 18-month check up, they described what had happened to him to their doctor. The doctor recommended testing by an allergist. The testing showed a severe peanut allergy and milder sensitivities to cashews and walnuts.

"Since that time, we have also seen a possible reaction begin when [he is] exposed to peanuts on someone else's breath. The only symptom of this possible reaction was crying (possible difficulty breathing), and he also ran and hid upon this exposure. This possible reaction subsided after a few minutes."

A True Allergy
Sensitivity to peanuts typically manifests itself in a true allergic reaction, sometimes a serious one that can include anaphylactic reaction.[45] And sensitivity to peanuts appears to be on the rise, perhaps because of its prevalence in so many forms in so many foods. Currently, it is believed that peanut allergy accounts for almost 30% of all food sensitivities, occurring most often in children under the age of 15 (who account for 93% of peanut allergy cases).[46] It's also believed that peanut allergy accounts for the majority of food related anaphylaxis deaths in the U.S.[47]

---

[45] Hourihane, Jonathan O'B, M.D. et al, Evaluation of the sensitivity of subjects with peanut allergy to very low doses of peanut protein: a randomized, double-blind, placebo-controlled food challenge study," Journal of Allergy and Clinical Immunology. November 1997
[46] Calgary Allergy Network.
[47] National Jewish Medical and Research Center, Denver, CO.

Peanuts, which are an inexpensive, readily available protein source, most often make their rounds as plain old peanut butter. But, according to the Asthma, Allergy, and Immunology Society of Ontario, they're making their way into more and more food products, directly, or through contamination from shared food preparation facilities.

While it's fairly well accepted that one reason for the increasing frequency and variety of food sensitivities Americans experience is due, in part, to frequent or repetitive exposure to those foods, peanuts dare to be different. In a 1989 study, 64% of children tested showed a positive RAST (indicating an allergy existed) to peanuts even though none of them had given a history of having eaten peanuts in the past. In one extreme example, a six-month-old baby had an anaphylactic reaction after eating a portion of a cracker containing peanut without ever having been previously exposed to peanuts. A subsequent RAST showed the child was highly sensitive to peanuts.[48]

Furthermore, a third of those allergic to peanuts are often allergic to tree nuts as well (although not necessarily other legumes, of which family peanuts are a member).[49] So it's strongly recommended that those demonstrating sensitivity to peanuts be tested for sensitivities to other nuts, as well. Conversely, if you or your child show sensitivity to tree nuts, it's wise to check to see if there's also a sensitivity to peanuts.[50]

Possible Sources
One factor in the supposed unpredictability of peanut sensitivity might be peanut consumption by expectant or breast-feeding mothers, suggests allergist Hugh Sampson and his colleagues at

---

[48] Weisnagel, John, M.D., "Peanut allergy: where do we stand?"

[49] See Food Families in Appendix.

[50] Calgary Allergy Network.

64

Mt. Sinai Medical School in New York.[51] These researchers believe that some problems can be avoided if foods known to cause sensitivities are not given to children in food sensitivity-prone families —via breast milk or otherwise—until the immune system has a chance to mature, usually between the ages of two and three. [52]

And while sensitivities to milk and egg may be outgrown, peanut allergy, like celiac disease, is typically life long. This is particularly difficult with peanuts, though, because so many foods are adulterated with it. Because of the inordinate difficulty in keeping peanuts out of the diet, and the severity of reactions associated with the sensitivity, several studies are underway to both understand the problem, and to find a way around it.

Hope for the Future
The National Jewish Medical and Research Center in Denver tested subjects with and without peanut sensitivity and discovered that T-cells (special cells that help fight infection and are involved in allergic responses) in both groups react to peanut protein. In those with known peanut sensitivities, though, their T-cells were unable to produce sufficient gamma interferon to inhibit that nasty allergy goblin, immunoglobulin E. They concluded that this means the T-cells in those sensitive to peanuts are abnormal, and they hope to be able to use this information to better study the sensitivity. [53]

Among possible treatments is "rush immunotherapy"—a series of steadily increasing injections of the allergy causing substance

---

[51] "Squires, Sally, "Increasing incidence of peanut allergy puts focus on food-reaction hazards, Outwitting allergens: Tips for eating safely," Washington Post, Oct. 23, 1996.

[52] Ibid.

[53] National Jewish Medical and Research Center: "New Peanut Allergy Development."

(in this case peanut extract) over a period of time. But the study is still in its infancy. And researchers at Mt. Sinai and the University of Arkansas have been working on the equivalent of a peanut allergy vaccine. But it, too, is only in the experimental stages.[54]

So, for now at least, knowing you or your child is allergic to peanuts means a dietary paradigm shift for life, i.e., the best treatment is complete avoidance of the allergenic substance. That means: *No peanuts*. This is a serious and severe sensitivity, wherein even trace amounts of the allergen can kill.

Anaphylactic Reactions
The most severe response to a food that an allergic person can have is an anaphylactic reaction. Anaphylactic reactions are nothing to fool with. They can begin suddenly, proceed quickly, and sometimes become fatal in a few minutes. Individuals most at risk must be treated immediately with epinephrine, which they must always keep nearby. The most common causes of anaphylaxis are food allergy, bee stings, and penicillin.

The symptoms of an anaphylactic reaction can include the following, any of which can lead to loss of consciousness, coma, and death:

- **Chills**
- **Runny nose**
- **Dizziness**
- **Itchy lips, mouth, eyes, tongue**
- **Gastrointestinal distress: vomiting, nausea, diarrhea**
- **Hives or flushed face**
- **Voice change**
- **Tightness in mouth, chest, or throat**
- **Rapid heartbeat**
- **Difficulty breathing or swallowing**
- **Feeling of impending doom**

---

[54] Bovsun, Mara, "Vaccine may prevent peanut allergy, " New York City, Washington, March 29 (UPI), MedServ Medical news, June 27, 1999.

It's worth repeating again that no one will be as careful or concerned about your children's health as you, so it's up to you to ensure your children's safety—especially the safety of the very young.

Never Assume Anything

"Never assume that other caregivers, teachers, etc., will always remember what they should do to provide safe food for your child, or what to do in case of an allergic reaction," warns Steve Kinsley. "You need to review the safety and emergency treatment measures with them periodically. We have found that many people, over time, almost forget that our son has a severe peanut sensitivity, or forget the signs of a reaction and what to do if a reaction does occur.

"When we think about the fact that, for the reactions our son had prior to being officially diagnosed, we did relatively little to deal with them (other than get very worried, but not call the hospital), we realize now that reactions should not be taken lightly. It's definitely best to respond quickly, even when you're not sure a reaction is really happening. An Epipen™[55] injection will not harm them (other than the needle pain) if a reaction is not actually happening. But if anaphylaxis is occurring, minutes can mean the difference between life and death." Also, experts recommend doing a "dry-run" with an EpiPen trainer device so you're prepared to use it correctly.

Know The Enemy...

As with all other sensitivities, but especially with something as potentially deadly as peanut allergy, it's important to educate both yourself and your child about the problem. In the case of peanut sensitivity, a certain amount of hyper-vigilance is in order, especially if your child is *severely* allergic to peanuts.

---

[55] EpiPen® is a commonly used brand of epinephrine. AnaGuard® is another common brand.

67

Peanut residues on counter tops can cause asthma in certain individuals. Even the odor of peanuts has been known to cause allergic reactions in highly sensitive individuals.

Peanuts are used in myriad ways, and are disguised under countless nom de plumes. Peanut butter can be used to thicken foods like chili, or to seal egg rolls. Peanuts can be altered and sold as other types of nuts. It's easy to contaminate baked goods or ice cream with peanuts. Some children may also have to avoid other legumes (the peanut family), including soy beans, peas, and garbanzo beans (chickpeas).[56]

Indeed, one of the biggest problems with peanut allergy is the insidious way peanuts have of cropping up out of nowhere—or seemingly from nowhere. The fact of the matter is that for those who are highly allergic to a substance, even a trace of that substance can cause a reaction. And since peanuts are used so often, in so many different foods and other preparations, cross-contamination is a major issue and one about which both families and children must be ever vigilant. Even something as benign as sitting in or touching a chair in which the previous person had left a trace of peanut residue can cause a reaction. For recent research on peanut allergies, see the Food Allergy Network's web site (www.foodallergy.org).

...And Keep Up With Him
Steve Kinsley, a registered dietitian who runs "NuConnexions," a diet software and resource company, [57] says the greatest challenge facing parents of children with peanut sensitivity is keeping up with food content.

---

[56] Allergy, Asthma and Immunology Society of Ontario
[57] See Resources in Appendix for contact information.

"… It is an ongoing challenge to keep this information up-to-date," says Kinsley. "We also find it very difficult to get others (especially other caregivers) to understand that just because an ingredient listing doesn't say, "may contain traces of nuts or peanuts", that doesn't mean that it will not contain traces, because it is not a legal requirement to put these warnings on food packaging. Many people assume that because they see these warnings on more foods, it must be a legal requirement to have it there (instead of just a voluntary measure by food companies).

Kinsley adds, "We have looked at the menus and products of daycare centers which are supposedly "peanut-free", but because of a lack of understanding of this labeling issue, we know that they are not truly "peanut-free". As a result, I look after my son while working from home, and when I have to work at a consulting client's office, we have him looked after by a friend who understands all the issues involved in providing safe food to our son."

Families with peanut allergic members must be extra careful about: using separate utensils to prepare foods, wrapping and storing foods separately, kissing and touching the sensitive child after possibly touching peanut-containing items, or even storing craft items in supposedly cleaned-out peanut butter jars. And, as always, everyone must excel at label reading.

Peanuts are in Asian sauces, in Italian pesto, in marzipan, in cakes, biscuits, bouillon, and Worcestershire® sauce. Many breakfast cereals contain peanuts. Hydrolyzed vegetable protein can be made of peanuts, as can lecithins. And, it's not just food or food additives—everyday toiletries like hand lotions and shampoos can contain peanut and other nut oils.

Eggs
A similar vigilance is in order for those sensitive to eggs. Like peanuts, eggs are one of the most highly allergenic of foods, and

69

even small amounts can cause reactions as severe as anaphylaxis. Also, as with peanuts, reactions can occur the very first
time that a sensitive individual is exposed to the allergen.[58] As
with most food sensitivities, the culprit in egg sensitivity is an
inability to digest certain proteins.

Proteins, Shmoteins
Eggs are made up of many proteins, but the four that cause the
most problems—ovomucoid, ovalbumin, ovotransfferin and
lysozyme—are found in egg whites and to a lesser extent egg
yolks. Of those, ovalbumin, which makes up half the egg white,
triggers the most reactions. But some people are allergic to egg
yolks, which contains a different set of equally unpronounced-
able proteins, namely apovitellenins I, apovitellenins VI, and
phosvitin (in case it comes up in a game of trivia.). Inhaled bird
antigens, resulting in some-thing called Bird Egg syndrome may
trigger egg yolk reactions.

And sometimes egg sensitivity can result from a cross-reaction
with seasonal environmental sensitivities, such as sensitivities
to oak pollen, ragweed, and goosefoot weeds.[59] In other words,
egg sensitivity can manifest itself in a variety of ways for a
variety of reasons, none of which make it any more comfortable
or easier to deal with than any other sensitivity.

Symptoms of Egg Sensitivity
Symptoms of egg sensitivity can include allergic rhinitis,
asthma, dermatitis, diarrhea and other gastrointestinal problems,
hives, nausea, vomiting, itching of the mouth and tongue,
wheezing and, at its most extreme, anaphylaxis. [60]

---

[58] Anderson, John A., M.D. "Milk, eggs and peanuts: food allergies in children, " American
Family Physician, Volume 56, No. 5, October 1, 1997.

[59] Ibid.

[60] Sicherer, Scott H., M.D., "Manifestations of food allergy: evaluation and management,"
American Academy of Family Physicians, January 15, 1999

Sharon knows right away when her daughter has been exposed to eggs. "If she eats egg she becomes wheezy, her nose runs, and sometime later she has diarrhea. If she eats quite a bit of egg the runny nose develops into what appears to be a cold followed by a chest infection. I have to avoid lecithin in her diet unless an ingredient specifically states soya lecithin as this affects her. The number of foods that contain eggs is amazing."

As with other sensitivities in children, sometimes behavioral problems can be traced to eggs. Barbara was concerned about her son's alternating moods. "The symptoms were tantrums, lack of reasoning, hitting, spitting, kicking—a most terrible child one minute, his calm self the next. The school system noticed he always had a bad Monday, and asked if there was anything we do on the weekend, that we do no other day. Every Sunday we ate eggs for breakfast at Grandma's house. We discontinued eggs (in everything) and found a whole new child."

Egg Hunt

Eggs, like peanuts, are masters of disguise. They're used frequently as binders, emulsifiers, and coagulants in foods, medicines and toiletries. They appear in baked goods (giving pretzels and cookies their shiny appearance), sauces, candy, processed meats, dairy products, pasta, soda, and cereal. They're also in lotions, shampoos, ointments, and vaccines[61] and in other pharmaceuticals.

And by now you know it's not as easy as just looking for "egg" on labels. If you're lucky, you'll find egg listed as egg white, egg white solids, egg yolk, powdered egg, etc. But most likely, egg

---

[61] John M. James, M.D., an allergist, points out that the current American Academy of Pediatrics Red Book 2000 recommends that patients with egg allergy, even those with severe histories of anaphylaxis to egg, may receive the measles, mumps, rubella (MMR) vaccine in the routine, one dose format.

71

will appear incognito as albumin, globulin, livetin, lysozyme, or lecithin (which can also be made with peanuts or soy) and all the proteins I mentioned before from both the whites and yolks.

Corn

Then there's the problem of corn sensitivity. This one can be particularly plaguing if you've been relying on corn as a substitute for wheat and then discover your child can't eat corn anymore either. As mentioned earlier, frequent exposure to any one food can create a sensitivity to it, which is why it's important to vary meals and ingredients as much as possible. Sometimes, though, you've just got a corn-sensitive individual on your hands. And then the solution, as always, is to eliminate corn from the diet. As with peanuts, eggs, milk, and wheat, that's easier said than done.

Corn Incognito

Corn sensitivity is most frequently expressed in skin rashes and asthma-like symptoms; again, the body's response to the proteins it is unable to digest. The good news is that at least corn oil is (usually) okay. During processing, the corn protein is removed, making it tolerable by most corn-sensitive people (although cold-pressed oils may not be totally protein-free).[62] But while it's easy to avoid obvious corn products like corn chips and tortillas, it's harder to avoid it as a hidden allergen in count-less foods that rely on cornstarch, cornmeal, and corn syrup as thickeners and sweeteners. Ingredients like dextrose can be made from corn, as can maltodextrin, and malt syrup. Dextrose of an unknown source can be used in everything from French fries to fish sticks, so, as usual, a great deal of diligence is in order if your child is sensitive to corn. Even caramel flavoring can be made with corn.

---

[62] Garriott, Linda, M.S., R.D., C.D.E., "Corn", Texas Department of Health and Michelle E. Morat, Texas A&M University, February 2000

Like peanuts and eggs before it, corn is also used frequently in places one might never expect to find it, from the adhesive in envelopes, stamps and stickers, to plastic wrap and paper cups and plates, although the latter are usually coated with corn oil, which usually causes no problems. It is even used in the processing of aspirin, ointments, vitamins and a variety of toiletry items, so it's important to know all its forms.

Again, the key is for you and your child to be both well educated about the problem and great label readers. Besides the obvious "corn" derivatives like cornstarch, corn meal or corn flour, and the dextrose ingredients, you have to be on the lookout for malt-type ingredients which can be made from corn.

Invert sugar, used in some candy and baked goods, is treated corn sugar. MSG is a famous corn derivative, known for producing unforgiving headaches in sensitive individuals. Any of the vague "vegetable-" ingredients, like vegetable protein, vegetable shortening, hydrolyzed vegetable protein and so forth, may contain corn.

And eating out can be a particular challenge for the corn sensitive. Chinese restaurants are best avoided, since cornstarch is a common thickener in Chinese food. Cold cuts are usually cured with a corn product. Almost all major soda brands are made with corn syrup, with the exception of diet sodas.

Soy
Although less allergenic than cow's milk, soy ranks 11th in allergenicity.[63] It is uncommon in adults (perhaps because they don't drink soy-based baby formulas very often!) and most—

---

[63] Hasler, Clare, Ph.D., Soy and Human Health Page at
<http://web.aces.uiuc.edu/faq.pdl?project_id=5&faq_id=331ag.uiuc.edu/~stratsoy/expert/askh ealth.html>

73

although not all—children outgrow soy sensitivity by age two. But it also appears to be on the rise.

According to the Allergy Society of South Africa, about one-fourth of cow-milk-sensitive patients become allergic to soy protein. John M. James, M.D., an allergist in private practice and board member of the Food Allergy Network, points that this figure is closer to 15% in the U.S.[64]

Soybean is often cited as one of the foods to which children experience IgE-mediated reactions. With its expanding use as a substitute and constituent in many different foods, a higher frequency of adverse reactions to soybean can be expected.

Symptoms of sensitivity to soy products include skin rashes, gastrointestinal problems, facial swelling, shortness of breath, difficulty swallowing, and possibly even anaphylactic reactions.

Once again, proteins are the culprits. At least 15 different proteins have been found in soy.[65] But soy sensitivity seems largely dependent on how the soy is processed. Fermented soy products like miso and tofu typically cause less sensitivity problems than raw soybeans.[66]

Because soy is an inexpensive, high protein food, it is used as the base for a lot of different prepared foods and label reading is essential if you're trying to get your toddler to that two year old stage where you hope he outgrows his soy sensitivity.

---

[64] John M. James, M.D., Personal Communication.

[65] Ogawa T. et al., "Investigation of the IgE-binding proteins in soybeans by imunoblotting with the sera of the soybean-sensitive patients with atopic dermatitis," Journal of Nutritional Science and Vitaminology. 1991; 37:555-565.

[66] Nelson, Roxanne, R.N., "How to Live With an Allergy to Soy", http:''www.ehow.com/eHow/eHow/0,1053, 3966, FF. html.

Sidestepping Soy

The essential task for the parent of a soy-sensitive toddler (or for that matter, for the older child or the stray soy-sensitive adult) is, of course, to completely eliminate soy from the diet. Even though some soy products may not cause a reaction, it's best to avoid all soy because it's difficult to evaluate the level of processing or safety of the food. This includes anything with hydrolyzed vegetable protein, textured soy protein, tofu, miso, okara, soy cheese, soy sauces, soy protein concentrates, isolates and flours, soy oil, tempeh, yuba, soy beverages, and possibly lecithin.[67] Mono and digylcerides, as well as mono-sodium glutamate may contain soy.

There is some debate about the safety of soy oil, since it can be produced without any of the soy protein in it—unless it's cold-pressed. The best rule of thumb here is, "*When it doubt, don't eat it.*" Seventy five percent of vegetable fats and oils in the U.S. come from soy. It's also used to make most margarines and vegetable shortenings, and is even found in dry lemonade mix.

And you have to ask a lot of questions when you eat out with a soy-sensitive child, since soy flour is often added to foods in restaurants for added protein, flavor, or thickening. It should go without saying that Chinese or Japanese restaurants probably wouldn't be a good choice for dinner, either.

Rice

Rice sensitivity strikes me as a sad thing to suffer, possibly because Chris likes it so much that it's hard not to make it a staple food around our house. Parting with rice would be as sorrowful as loosing those Cheerios™. Rice is beautiful. You can make artwork with all the colors and shapes it comes in! It's

---

[67] Hasler: Soy and Human Health Page.

75

delicious and malleable, a culinary marvel that lends itself to a seemingly endless variety of dishes.

It bespeaks an entire culture; it's eaten every single day in Eastern Asia. And, consequently, it's the most common food sensitivity there, and relatively rare in the U.S. and Europe. Rice sensitivity is often closely associated with grass pollen sensitivities, as well. It's also more common in adults than children, one might presume because of their long-term exposure to rice. [68]

Symptoms of rice sensitivity include mostly skin rashes, some gastrointestinal disturbances, asthma and, sometimes, anaphylaxis. Although this is largely a problem of adulthood, and more common outside the U.S. and Europe, it's important to consider rice as a possible allergen, especially since cross-reactivity with other grains is sometimes in evidence.[69] And it's an important reminder that an unvaried diet, with frequent exposure to a limited number of foods can result in sensitivity to those foods.

Other Problematic Foods

There are also some lesser known, but equally problematic food sensitivities. Anaphylactic reactions to potatoes have been found, although it's believed that the allergen in this case is largely the skin of the potato.[70] Those sensitive to potatoes must also be careful about handling or being touched by (as in a medical care situation) natural rubber latex. Latex can produce sometimes severe cross-reactions known as "latex-fruit syndrome". Foods most often affecting latex-allergic patients are avocado, banana, chestnut, and kiwi, although the Food Allergy

---

[68] Internet Symposium on Food Allergens 1(4): 147-60 (1999)

[69] Nakase M, Usui Y, Alvarez-Nakase AM, Adachi T, Urisu A, Nakamura R, Aoki N, Kitajima K, Matsuda T (1998), "Cereal allergens: rice-seed allergens with structural similarity to wheat and barley allergens," Allergy 53(46 Suppl.): 55-7

[70] Potatoes, along with tomatoes and peppers are members of the nightshade family, and sensitivities to one often entail sensitivities to related foods. See Food Families in Appendix.

Network also lists papaya, passion fruit, fig, melon, mango, pineapple, peach, and tomato.[71]

Multiple Sensitivities

Sometimes, children suffer from multiple sensitivities, making their diet a challenge for even the most organized of parents. Andrew is one of those children.

Cindy's Story

"We suspected our son had food allergies at about seven or eight months. Shortly after we started him on first foods for babies, we noticed he would break out in hives after every meal. The hives wouldn't usually last for long, maybe an hour. But it seemed that whatever we tried eliminating from his diet, he still broke out. After taking him to an allergist, he tested positive for 21 foods," says Cindy.

Among Andrew's sensitivities were sensitivities to all legumes, rice, egg, pork, potato, shellfish, and peanut. His problems manifested themselves more in colitis-like symptoms, says Cindy. "[He had] frequent constipation, stomach cramps, and hemorrhoids. I have noticed with the improvement of his food sensitivities, and with abstaining from the foods he is allergic to, that his colitis is basically non-existent, with just the occasional problem of slight bleeding from hard stool." Now, at the grand old age of 3 1/2, Andrew is down to sensitivities to just five foods: pork, potato, peanut, shellfish and egg.

Going largely on their allergist's conviction that "with complete avoidance of the allergen, the body stops producing antibodies

---

[71] Brehler-R; et al, "Latex-fruit syndrome: frequency of cross-reacting IgE antibodies, European Journal of Allergy and Clinical Immunology, April, 1997 For an excellent discussion on latex allergies, see *Food Allergy and Latex Allergy: Is There A Connection* in The Food Allergy Network's newsletter, Food Allergy News, (Volume 9, No.5, June-July 2000). By the way, this article adds grapes and apricots to this list.

against that allergen," Andrew's family eliminated all the problem foods from his diet and met with considerable success.

"We made sure that A.J. ate absolutely none of his allergens. And our doctor tested him once a year. The first couple of years he had improvement each time. Now with his last tests, he remained the same for foods, so he won't be tested again for two years. The doctor feels he has sort of hit a plateau, and that there is no reason to put him through the tests for a little while. But I hope that eventually he will be at least almost sensitivity free. He has the peanut and shellfish allergies, which doctors don't feel there is a very good chance of overcoming."

Barbara, who met with such success when she took eggs from her son's diet, later discovered other problems. "The summer he was five, we discovered he loved my iced tea. We started seeing the awful, uncontrollable child again, and knew it was the tea," Barbara said.

"More home testing revealed that caffeine, rather than the tea, was the cause. We had him sensitivity-tested with needle pricks. Wheat was taken off the list, (a big plus), tree pollen, nuts and other allergens were found. A substantial sensitivity to milk and eggs was confirmed."

Juliann's Story
Juliann has two children with multiple food sensitivities. Her now four-year-old son, John, has confirmed sensitivities to barley, milk, soy, peanuts, nuts, legumes, chocolate, eggs, salmon, and possibly to BHA, BHT, TBHQ[72], nitrites or sulfites. Her two-year-old daughter, Cathy, is sensitive to corn, chocolate and salicylate (citrus, spices, mints, and berries).

---

[72] Butylated hydroxyanisole (BHA), and butylated hydroxytoluene (BHT) and tertiary butylhydroquinone (TBHQ) are antioxidant additives that slow the oxidation and consequent spoilage of prepackaged foods.

78

They discovered her son's problems when they tried giving him soy formula as a baby. "I nursed, so John usually didn't have formula. We tried soy formula (since we already knew he had milk problems). He wouldn't even drink it. When he finally drank 1 oz, within an hour or two, his temperature shot up to 104° F. About a year later (at around 20 months of age), he stopped growing and dropped below the 5% height curve (he started at 95%). We got a RAST blood test, which was a godsend, and [it] told us about barley, which he craved, among other allergies. The test wasn't completely accurate, as eggs showed up negative, though we knew he had reactions to eggs. We stopped his bi-weekly Chinese restaurant soy sauce ingestion and his chronic night time coughing stopped."

Her infant daughter's initial problems were solved by adjustments to Juliann's diet. "When I worked and nursed Cathy in the evenings, she would wake up consistently at 1 am. I learned that it was due to my eating some lunchmeat (at noon that day) which contained corn syrup."

Again, a major tenet of dealing with any of these food sensitivities, including multiple sensitivities, is to stay on top of things at all times.

Cover All Your Bases
"When eating out," says Kinsley, "Ask very explicit questions of the restaurant owners regarding the safety of the food for your child who has a peanut (or other) food sensitivity. "In any setting where your child is cared for by others and receives food of any kind, including not only daycare, but also things like church nurseries and Sunday schools, make sure the caregivers understand the food sensitivity issue. And try to get all possible snacks and food provided to all children to be safe from a food sensitivity perspective. Remember, children often spontaneously share food in these settings."

79

And with multiple children with multiple sensitivities, there's no substitute for organization either. "With two kids having different allergies," says Juliann, "I code their food with stickers or marker. One gets reinforcements (circles) while the other gets dots. Foods that have not been tried are labeled 'test'."

She also keeps extensive records and files all her information where others in the family can find it. Then, in the event that anything should happen to her, says Juliann, "my spouse or another has an immediate resource to information that took me years to compile."

She also suggests keeping a "Sensitivities vs. Allowed Foods" list. "Distribute copies to the doctor, daycare, (and) relatives. Keep one posted at home so your spouse and sitters can use it."

Stay Informed
The old adage, "Never assume anything" is never more appropriate than when dealing with food sensitivity, as Steve Kinsley points out so well.

"Never assume that just because a particular food product was once safe from a food sensitivity perspective, that it will remain so. Periodically check with the companies. This is especially true for products prepared for grocery store chains by other companies—the companies contracted to do this for the grocery store chains tend to change over time, but the packaging may not change to indicate this. "

Make It Yourself
Usually the best solution is the most obvious. *Make it Yourself.* "If you have the time and ability," says Cindy, "make it homemade. That way you are sure what is going into it."

Barbara agrees. "I cook mostly from scratch—no boxed or frozen meals. It is much less expensive, even though the

80

individual ingredients cost more than the standard shelf stock sometimes."

And making an effort to fix meals and treats that are safe for your child but that friends and family can enjoy goes a long way towards feelings of inclusiveness and comfort for the food-sensitive child. Barbara goes the extra step to provide her son's daycare center with foods she has prepared ahead of time, which they can refrigerate or freeze there for him.

"When another child brings in cupcakes for a birthday to share, my son's just come out of the freezer to thaw, so he can have one when the rest of the class does."

And home prepared foods and meals needn't be complicated or time consuming. Keeping it simple can keep it just as safe—and make it more routine—than a lot of involved kitchen work. Simply cooked, lightly seasoned vegetables, allowed grains, greens and salads, fruits, lean meats and poultry—all within your child's safety zone of edibles of course—make perfectly tasty, pleasant meals the whole family can enjoy.

Make It a Family Affair
"We work very hard at making all the foods we love, in such a way that everyone in the family can eat them," says Barbara.

Cindy agrees that it's important for children with special diets not to feel left out. "We have altered our diets and recipes so that we all eat what my son can have. That way, at least in his own home, he can have everything that everyone else has."

Also, the easier you make feeding your child, the more your child can help with his own diet and the earlier he can become empowered to manage it with self-confidence, culinary grace and accuracy. "As children grow, they must be taught how to

81

deal with their situation with a positive mental attitude," says Barbara. "We can't do this so let's do that, kind of idea."

And with the paradigm shift required of embarking on special diets for life, comes a certain epiphany, unexpected blessings of sorts, says Juliann. "Life is simpler," she says of their " back to basics, cook from scratch" lifestyle. "Maybe we'll live healthier, without all the additives common in foods today. "I have been chosen to take care of this special child," she adds. "And (I have been) called to use my abilities and resources to their fullest. In doing so, I will change and grow into a more rounded and better person."

Barbara reminds us that this will be a "lifetime project" for some children. Something as simple as letting them help in the kitchen now will give them skills they can use later, and the confidence to deal with the next big issue facing families and their food-sensitive children: Well-meaning family and friends.

Summing It All Up

- *Symptoms of a food allergy may include:*
  - Allergic rhinitis
  - Asthma
  - Dermatitis, eczema
  - Difficult swallowing
  - Gastrointestinal disturbance
  - Itching of mouth, tongue
  - Shortness of breath
  - Anaphylaxis
  - Diarrhea
  - Facial swelling
  - Hives
  - Nausea and vomiting
  - Skin rashes
  - Wheezing

- *Peanut allergy accounts for almost 30% of all food reactions, occurring most often in children under the age of 15, who account for 93% of all peanut allergy cases.*
  - Peanut allergy is believed to account for the majority of food-related anaphylaxis deaths in the U.S.
  - Peanut allergy is typically not outgrown.
  - Peanut allergy can occur with no previous exposure.

- **Anaphylactic reaction to peanuts can include:**
  - Chills
  - Dizziness
  - Hives or flushed face
  - Runny nose
  - Voice change
  - Rapid heartbeat
  - Itchy lips, mouth, eyes, or tongue
  - Gastrointestinal distress: vomiting, nausea, diarrhea
  - Difficulty breathing or swallowing
  - Tightness in mouth, chest, or throat

- *Eggs, like peanuts, are one of the most highly allergenic foods* —small amounts can cause anaphylactic reactions. As with peanuts, reactions can occur during the very first exposure.

- *Other food sensitivities include*:
  - *Corn sensitivity is most frequently expressed in skin rashes and asthma*, the body's response to proteins it can't digest.
  - *Soy ranks 11th in allergenicity.* It is uncommon in adults and most—although not all—children outgrow soy sensitivity by the age of two.
  - *Rice sensitivity (relatively rare in the U.S.)* is the most common food sensitivity in Eastern Asia, where rice is eaten daily. It is often closely associated with grass pollen sensitivities, as well, and is more common in adults than in children. Cross-reactivity with other grains sometimes occurs.

- *Some children have multiple food sensitivities, but patients with true food allergies are rarely allergic to more than two foods.* Be sure to keep records for each child's diet where others can find them.

- *Safeguard your child's health and well-being.* Whether your child suffers from one food sensitivity or many, it's important to:
  - Excel at label reading
  - Know the various names and forms of food ingredients
  - Prepare as many foods as possible for your child yourself.
  - Empower your child early on, by making him familiar with

83

foods he can eat and how to prepare them

- **Keep It Simple and Safe with easy to fix meals and snacks the whole family can enjoy together.**

Part II

Food Sensitive and Free:
Making Team Members of Family, Friends, Caregivers, and Peers

Chapter V
Family, Friends, and Caregivers:
"Grandma's Not Trying to Kill You, She Just Doesn't Know What Gluten Is (or Casein, or ...)"

Relatives, especially close ones like grandparents, scoffed or thought we were being over-protective when we opted for Chris' healthy new wheat-free diet. Who in their right mind, they wondered, would take away the most fundamental part of a child's diet, the staff of life, the source of all nutrition since the beginning of time?! God threw bread from the sky, for goodness sakes! It just *can't* be bad for him, they argued.

"Children NEED bread," a concerned relative told me. "Poor child!"

That seemed to be the overwhelming consensus. "Poor Chris!" How would he ever live without bread? Without cookies? Without a plate of chicken fried steak or Kentucky Fried Chicken™? If Chris had been older, these plaintive cries on his behalf would quite likely have made it more difficult for him to endure his dietary change. But we usually did our best to have him out of earshot when the family protests began—and they were frequent in those early months.

Constantly, one of his grandmothers would hand him a cookie or a slice of bread. He would hand it back, almost apologetically. "I can't. I'm 'lergic," he would say in his tiny voice over and over again. Sometimes he'd look at me hopefully and ask, "Right?" And I'd reassure him that he was indeed right and remind him of his discomfort when he ate wheat.

85

"Grandmom's not trying to hurt you," I'd reassure him. "She just doesn't know what gluten is." And that was really the long and the short of it. No one realized the prevalence of wheat in our daily diet. In our world of prepackaged convenience foods, we had stopped looking at labels—other than for saturated fat content and calories—and forgotten that nearly all prepackaged foods are made of numerous ingredients. Even the most recognized of foods had lost their significance as having a grain-based source. They just were what they were, as if divinely created in a box.

Our family was incensed that I wouldn't give him spaghetti, forgetting, of course, that spaghetti is skinny wheat. "How about a graham cracker?" my mother asked. "What's graham flour?" I asked in return. "Oh," came the crestfallen reply.

We were inundated with well-meaning but erroneous advice and boxes of snack foods people thought were safe, but were chock full of "food starch" or "wheat" or "wheat gluten". All were intestinal death sentences for Chris. Constantly, we pointed out villains on the sides of boxes. Constantly, eyes rolled at us. But gradually, with patience and persistence, what became routine for us gained acceptance by the rest of the family.

We discovered, as Lindsay pointed out, that the key to that acceptance was to " Educate, educate, and educate again anyone who provides your child with food."

The Three Point Plan
It's a three-point education program. First, you need to be educated yourself, about all the aspects of your child's food sensitivity, as well as about your child's environment. How much of that environment can you control? How much can you trust others on whom you must rely when you're not physically with your child? How well do others understand the issue? Do they even care?

86

Second, you need to start educating your child as soon as possible, so that he or she is in control as early as possible. The goal isn't to make your child afraid of his sensitivity, but comfortable and confident controlling it.

And third, you need to educate everyone around you—family, friends, daycare providers, or teachers—who come into daily contact with your child.

The point is you can't leave anything to chance when you're dealing with a food sensitivity, and you certainly can't abdicate your responsibility where your child's health is concerned. It's up to you to have all your bases covered.

> *"It is very important for people to understand there is always a new food allergy that you may not know about so don't dismiss a child or mother like they don't know what they are talking about. It makes things very difficult."*
> —Edith's daughter

That means you have to educate and empower your child as much as possible, provide food when and where necessary, and carefully choose and educate the people who will take care of your child when you're not around.

A High Wire Act
In the early years, it's a balancing act of organized involvement in your child's activities at school or daycare, enlisting the advocacy of caring friends, relatives, daycare providers, and teachers, and reinforcing positive eating habits and educated responses in your child as soon as he can talk.

Using some allergy management guidelines compiled from the Food Allergy Network (FAN), the Allergy Awareness Association in New Zealand, the American Academy of Allergy, Asthma and Immunology (AAAAI), the American College of Allergy, Asthma, and Immunology (ACAAI), and the International Food Information Council (IFIC), and a variety of other sources, let's look at who you should educate, how you should educate them, and what else you can do to help your food-sensitive children and the adults in their lives work towards the same, healthy ends.

Assemble Your Team
- **Make your immediate family your child's primary support team.**
-

Touchingly, your child's first major ally, besides you, will be a sibling. That became the case as we dealt with Chris' food sensitivities from quite early on. His older sisters, at the ripe old age of three and five, became his guardian angels and royal food tasters.

"Should he eat that, Mommy?" One or the other of them would ask me. They'd read labels right beside me in the grocery store, scan menus seriously and one of my daughters has become quite adroit at detecting seasoning in French fries and other foods, which may indicate wheat flour was used in the preparation of the food.

Other families report similar experiences. "My four year old is conscious of Sam's diet and is quick to tell me when Sam has something I haven't given him," reports Lindsay." He also tells others feeding Sam. He has taken both my mom and the daycare provider to task when he thought they were giving Sam something they shouldn't."

"I don't want Joe to feel responsible for his brother's diet so I never mention it to him unless he asks. But I do compliment him for being aware, asking questions, and intervening when he does. The fact is, Joe can be very helpful until Sam can manage on his own and I appreciate that but don't want to burden Joe."

Karen's practically deputized Cody's siblings. "We were in Wal-Mart one day and there was a popcorn testing booth. My older son, who was six at the time, asked the lady in the booth if the popcorn was gluten free. The poor lady didn't have a clue what he was asking about so I helped out. Cody's older brother and sister have been real good as "gluten police" for their younger brother."

Include Everyone

All of these are ideal scenarios: the entire immediate family, parents and siblings, acting as a guiding force of health and well-being around the food-sensitive child still too young to manage his own choices. But it doesn't come without effort, and without attention to the needs of non-food-sensitive members of the family. If the world revolves around the food-sensitive child, there's a danger of creating bitterness and jealousy among others. But if food is treated as simply one aspect of everyone's life, without placing undue emphasis upon what any one person may or may not eat, then no one will be singled out as "special" or "different," labels you want to avoid at home as much as elsewhere.

When Cindy makes sure there's something for her celiac son on special occasions, she also ensures that her non-food-sensitive daughter isn't short-changed. "Sometimes it is hard, because it seems unfair to not allow my daughter some of her favorite treats, just because my son can't have them. We find it safer all the way around for his allergens to not be in the house. But when we are out, I allow my daughter to get her favorites, and make sure that my son can have something special that is also safe for him."

☑ **Before the school year begins, schedule a meeting with your child's teachers, school administrators, counselor, nurse, cafeteria personnel and office staff. Explain to this "team" what foods cause a reaction, precautions, emergency procedures, how to read a label and lunch time considerations. Have the same kind of meeting with family or friends who will be caring for your child.**

89

The word "team" is a good one to use. Everyone who works with children, from family and friends to daycare and school personnel are part of any child's advocacy team. No one questions the fact that these daily children's teams are responsible for the health and safety of the children in their care.

For Lee, the school nurse is the head of her son Jimmy's "team." "The school nurse has been my most important ally—she has advocated for Jimmy, investigated the ingredients in 'snack bar' items, and just been there for him and for me," she says. And that has been an enormous help and a big relief for Jimmy's family.

The Law is on Your Side

Ideally, if parents have done their part, helping a child maintain a special diet should present caregivers no greater obstacle to ensuring health and safety than keeping children safe in a playground. And, caregivers also have a commensurate legal responsibility to ensure your child's dietary safety. Section 504 of the Rehabilitation Act of 1973, the Individuals with Disabilities Education Act (IDEA) of 1997 Public Law 105-17, was signed by President Clinton on June 4, 1997. The Final IDEA '97 Regulations were released in March of 1999[73].

The law provides for "supplementary aids and services" for children having "limited strength, vitality, and alertness," for a variety of reasons including chronic or acute health problems that "adversely affects a child's educational performance." That means that schools must make every effort to provide your child's education in an environment that's safe and free of impediments to his or her learning, in relation to his or her problem, be it physical or emotional.

---

[73] You can obtain a copy of this law from the Superintendent of Documents, U.S. Gov. Printing Office, P.O. Box 371954, Pittsburgh, PA 15250-7954. Or, access the entire act, with links by topic, online at http://www.ideapractices.org/lawandregs.htm

Specifically, the IDEA Amendments of 1997 promise to "Preserve the right of children with disabilities to a free appropriate public education" by doing these things:
- Strengthen the role of parents
- Focus on teaching, and learning while reducing unnecessary paperwork requirements;
- Ensure schools are safe and conducive to learning; and
- Encourage parents and educators to work out their differences by using non-adversarial means.

In addition, the Free Appropriate Public Education portion of the law (§300.532) says that evaluation procedures must "provide that each child's evaluation must be sufficiently comprehensive to identify all of the child's special education and related services needs".

All of that is to say that, if all else fails during your team building efforts, there are statutory measures in place to protect your child in school if need be. The IDEA ensures that your food-sensitive child has access to his or her special foods, to medications, and to safe activities. More than likely, you'll never need to call upon the Individuals with Disabilities Education Act to make sure your child is safe in school. But when you're free-falling through a food sensitivity, it's reassuring to know you've got a reserve chute.

Keep it in Perspective
Now you certainly don't want to go the other way and insist that everything revolve around your child. One allergy fact sheet suggested: "For class parties, you may want to request that all parents avoid sending foods containing substances that may cause an allergic reaction (this may also be a permanent request for school lunches)." You can certainly try to make such a request, but you have to ask yourself if that's a reasonable request. There could be a myriad other food sensitivities in your child's classroom besides your child's alone. And is that even fair to the other children? Will that create resentment in them in their future treatment of your child?

91

Remember that the idea here is to help your child become a regular part of his or her society—to *eat differently without seeming different*—and you can't do that by making everyone treat your child as sublimely special. What you want to do is create a safe, secure environment in which your child can interact with others as easily and conveniently as possible. The burden for much of that seamless interaction lies on you for a while, and then eventually is passed to your child.

More than a Mealtime Issue

Make sure caregivers also understand that the problem can go beyond meal issues alone. Go over proposed classroom or daycare activities with teachers and caregivers to evaluate craft, art or cooking projects for safety. Celiac children playing with traditional play dough can ingest the dough either directly, or by rubbing their face or eyes during play, and the gluten in the play-dough can provoke a reaction. Children with peanut or egg sensitivities can have reactions if either ingredient is used for crafts or cooking projects.

Using milk containers or milk lids for various projects can create problems for children with milk sensitivities. Residues left on tables and chairs can be allergenic as well. Be sure caregivers and teachers know when they can rely on you to help in classroom activities, and be prepared to suggest or provide materials such as alternative containers of gluten-free play dough[74] when you feel that might be helpful.

Also, discuss possible field trips with administrators and teachers, and be sure they know to contact you before taking your child on any possible food-related trip. Children with egg allergy could have a reaction visiting a bakery where egg powder might be airborne; not to mention the vigilance required for keeping bread samples out of the hands of wheat-sensitive kids. Visiting a candy or nut factory might create problems for those with peanut or tree nut sensitivities. If at all possible,

---

[74] See Chapter 11 for gluten-free play dough.

92

chaperone during trips to minimize work for teachers and worry for yourself.

The Learning Curve
Sam's daycare was a serious issue for Lindsay. "Because they saw him so ill, we never went through that "one little cookie can't hurt him" thing. But there was a learning curve, especially for the daycare provider to get up to speed on the diet."

Everyone has that learning curve regarding special diets. It's one thing to accept that a child (or an adult for that matter) has a food sensitivity. It's quite another for people to learn to respect it, along with all its accompanying issues. Lynda's husband, for instance, accepts his son's condition, said Lynda, but "He doesn't understand how many faces this disease has—contamination issues, behavioral concerns, other medical conditions, social isolation, etc."

Part of the problem is that there is rarely any real "outward" sign of a problem in those with food sensitivities. "People take an 'allergy' seriously if they think a child will go into anaphylactic shock," Tracey notes. "But it's hard to take something seriously if you don't see a reaction." And kids older than toddlers often aren't eager to share information about their delayed reactions with others.

Draw Good Pictures
Sometimes you have to resort to using comparisons that doubters can relate to better. Almost everybody knows someone with a food-related illness, even though they may not even realize it. Diabetes is one of the best examples for the dubious. Most people are willing to accept that diabetes requires dietary management and even medical treatment. Try explaining that food sensitivities are much the same thing. The body has an improper reaction to food that causes illness and discomfort and, sometimes, behavioral problems. And the best way to eliminate those problems is to avoid the food that causes them.

93

It doesn't get much simpler than that! Keep some good, easy to read medical discussions on hand to share (there are good references in the Appendix.)

With the more deadly issue of anaphylaxis in relation to peanut or egg allergy, you have to be firm and insistent. Explain precisely what an anaphylactic reaction is; relate it to snake bite, bee stings, poisoning, anything you think will get your point across on the danger of ingesting the forbidden food. This is particularly important if you're dealing with relatives who will be acting as caretakers in your absence, or with daycare providers.

Once you feel the true nature of the problem is understood by those involved:

☑ *Enable Your Team. Make it as easy as possible for team members to give you the help you need.*

The more information you can keep in the right hands, the better. Consider yourself your child's health librarian until he or she has the required knowledge base to educate others alone. In addition to teaching your child's team what foods are safe for your child, make sure they know what type of reaction your child might have if the wrong food is eaten. You might try to get team members to watch "*It Only Takes One Bite*," or both team members and peers to view "*Alexander, the Elephant Who Couldn't Eat Peanuts,* " both available from the Food Allergy Network (FAN).[75] FAN also produces an excellent pamphlet called "*Off to School With Food Allergies*" that caretakers will benefit from reading.

---

[75] Order from Food Allergy Network, 10400 Eaton Place, Suite 107, Fairfax, VA 22030, or online at http://foodallergy.org/. FAN also carries a big line of literature, films, posters, and guides for helping families and children understand and deal with food sensitivities in a variety of situations and settings. See their new web site for kids at <http://fankids.org>.

If your child needs epinephrine injections for a severe food allergy, make sure caregivers are trained in its use and practice a few times to be comfortable giving the injection. Make sure all involved parties have epinephrine on hand, and an accompanying instruction booklet for using it.

Provide Lots of Information and Keep It Everywhere
Also provide all "team members" with a form like the one Food Allergy Survivors Together (FAST) has created. The "Contact Form" for children is reprinted in the Appendix as a reproducible master, and helps you provide complete and detail-ed information for anyone who might need it. Make copies for everyone—preferably on brightly colored paper to make it especially hard to miss, and one on white paper in case they need to make additional copies. And keep an extra copy handy to show to or leave with any substitute caregivers. Look the form over regularly and revise it as needed. Ask your doctor to complete a medical information form for your child, as well. And highlight all allergy information in bright ink on all forms to make sure no one misses vital information.

Consider laminating a miniaturized version of your child's Contact Form and attaching it to schoolbags, putting it in your child's wallet or attaching it to clothing. And, of course, Medic Alert® bracelets or necklaces are always good reminders. "We bought Sam a Medic Alert® bracelet," Lindsay says. "More to remind people who already know about his diet to think of it as a "top of the mind" issue when food is around. It's been helpful and Sam will tell people who ask about the bracelet, "No gluten for Sam". We think this is a good start for a two year old..."

Make Food Sensitivities a "Top of the Mind" Issue
Keeping it a "top of the mind" issue is the trick. Complacency can be the biggest enemy of the food-sensitive. So the easier you make it for those whose help you and your child need, the easier it will be for them to take care of your child in a safe and

95

appropriate manner. And the best way to do that, Barbara reminds us again, is to never assume anything.

"Don't presume when you tell someone your child has ... an allergy that they understand how to avoid things that cause symptoms," says Barbara. "If your child might have a reaction when you are not around (daycare or overnight at Grandma's), make sure they have something written down as to what the symptoms are, and what they should do. These mini-emergencies do not trigger automatic responses in people who are not familiar with them.

"I mention 'if your child might have a reaction.' Occasionally, you know when he ate something he shouldn't have. You don't anticipate a reaction strong enough to keep him home from daycare that day. But daycare providers must know, if he becomes uncomfortable, what to do and when it is serious enough to call you or take some other action."

Sam's family and long time caretakers have first hand knowledge of his reactions, Lindsay says, so they don't try to sneak in treats they've been told aren't safe. "At this point they do well with it but that is always a nagging worry I have."

Hedge Your Bets
It's hard to overcome that nagging worry. That's probably a good thing. It keeps us on our toes. But again, the easier you make it for everyone else—by providing written instructions regarding the proper action to take in case of a reaction, by bringing and storing appropriate foods where your child will be taken care of away from home and by educating everyone as much as possible, the less that worry will nag you.

Lindsay even hedges her dietary bets with computer assistance, the results of which she can share all the way around. "My best tool to manage his diet is the Excel database I have put together from products I have called about or learned are gluten free. I

96

used the Tri-Counties[76] guide as a starter and then pared it down to only products we use and added what I found from the Internet list [and elsewhere]. I am very careful with Sam's diet and don't take many risks with products. So I try to update each year or more, and don't take every product claimed as gluten-free on a listserve as a definitive."

"…Each time I update I give a copy to grandma, the caregiver and keep one in the diaper bag as well as my home/grocery store copy. I also added a page for restaurants so I know what to order."

☑ **Keep and maintain a supply of snacks at your child's school or caregiver's or other family members' homes.**

This is also a great way to start getting across that "healthy birthright" concept. The more healthy snacks and foods you can prepare and provide for your child in other environments, the more accepting others will be and the more integrated your child's involvement with others will be.

"Keep things your child *loves* always on hand for times when they can't have what everyone else is having," says Barbara. "We always keep M&M's™, Dietary Specialties™ pretzels, raisins, and gluten-free cookies in the diaper bag so we are never caught without options."

Talk to your child's daycare or preschool about their openness to your providing your child's foods there on a regular basis. Carefully mark your child's foods and describe each item to his caregivers. Do the same for family and friends. Keep special foods for your child in specially marked containers at homes where your child stays often. Provide lists of appropriate substitutes, with instructions to contact you before any substitutions are made. Remind caregivers of young children's

---

[76] TriCounties Shopping List ordering information is in the Appendix under Celiac Sprue Resources.

penchant for sharing their food, and if at all possible, try to make sure as much of the food used in social situations is allergen free.

Be Patient
It's also important to remember that, just as it's easy for *us* to forget our children's problems when gluten free or dairy free is a home time routine, it's even easier for others to forget they need to provide for those problems when they don't have to deal with them daily. If it's not something you do all the time, it's going to seem strange and difficult. Remembering that can help you be patient and understanding with family and friends. Just remember, the easier you make it for others to help you and your child, the more willingly they will.

"I don't trust anyone who doesn't cook for Sam on a daily basis to cook occasionally," says Lindsay. "I just feel there are too many hidden complications. So I call before we go over and coach them on what they could prepare gluten-free and I know what to supplement by bringing. I sent my product list to family members we spend extended holidays with and they shopped from that so there were gluten-free options in the house."

Karen simply sends Cody to special occasions with his own version of C.A.R.E packages. For school parties or special occasions, she says, " I make some cupcakes and Cody takes a couple with him. If they are having pizza I send a personal size one they can warm up in the oven (it fits in a pie plate so nothing will touch it). If they are having hotdogs I send those and a bun that can be nuked in the microwave. He has never been left out of his friends parties."

Get Involved
☑ **Be prepared to be involved in your child's daycare, preschool, or school activities.**

98

Expect to be chaperone, teacher's assistant, den mother, scout leader or all of the above at a lot of events for a while!

"Get involved in everything your celiac child is involved in so you can influence the food decisions," says Janet. "Our rule has been to keep Michael's life as normal as possible. This has meant a tremendous effort on our part, but has worked well. I have baked for every single school party, scouting event, and church event so that there is gluten-free food for Michael. I always made whole batches so that the other kids were eating the same thing as Michael and he wasn't singled out by having special food. When there are pizza or hotdog parties, I just bring his and heat it up separately."

Sometimes, caregivers' best intentions can go awry, and then patience and understanding are important. If you're consistently involved and familiar with your children's caretakers, you can usually intervene and correct any problems fairly quickly.

One of Cody's teachers went to great efforts to learn about celiac disease, recalls Karen. "She read the Celiac Disease Handbook (a local resource guide) cover to cover when I took it in on Cody's first day of school."

"I think that if someone tells you that they have a food allergy look into it before you call them a liar. It can hurt their feelings, making it more difficult for the person with the allergy to cope with it and make them very confused, frustrated, and/or angry with you. In the long run it will make them trust you more and you will have a better knowledge of certain food allergies."
—Jane

Another teacher, though, just tried to wing it. "She would phone and say that she had bought some Rice Krispie treats for Cody since they were having a celebration at school the next day and she had seen Cody eating them before. I would remind her again that Cody's Rice Krispie treats[77] were homemade with special ingredients and that I would send extra cookies or treats for their celebration."

The more involved you are, the less you have to leave to chance, and the more you contribute to your child's sense of safety and belonging.

"I became a class mother," says Lee," and put together a simple list of snack foods (complete with brand name) that are safe for Jimmy. Involvement is the answer! And Jim is so thrilled that his Mom plans the parties and everything!"

When children in a class bring in special treats for some occasion, have your child provide fruit trays or gluten-free trail mixes that everyone can enjoy. Sometimes, you can bake treats for a day care center or preschool to freeze for your child and thaw during special occasions like birthdays or holiday celebrations. This is also a good way to provide impromptu education for others about food and health. Always remember to say "thank-you" to those who go out of their way to help your child.

Empowerment

☑ **Empower your child by promoting healthy caution instead of debilitating fear.**

Teach your child all about his or her food sensitivity, at whatever level you feel your child can understand. Explain what foods cause a reaction and the importance of avoiding them for his own comfort and well-being. Talk about more serious medical problems that affect others, and be positive and upbeat about your child's food sensitivities, pointing out how fortunate it is that the problem can be solved by diet alone.

---

[77] Kellogg's Rice Krispies®, the most commonly found, have the ingredient "malt" in them, which is a wheat derivative and should be avoided by those on gluten-free diets. A gluten-free version of this traditional treat is in Chapter 11.

Be Supportive

Children can be extremely reluctant to report a reaction to a particular food, especially if they fear discipline or a strong parental reaction. In the event your child does eat the wrong thing, instead of scolding, help your child feel better and, at a more appropriate time, discuss what happened and whether or not it was an accident. If your child sneaked something he shouldn't have, remind him that ultimately, his health and well-being will be his responsibility.

If it was an accident, remember that accidents happen and you can both try to be more vigilant next time. But a matter of fact approach to the event will do more to create confidence and trust than nagging and chastising.

"I've met one child who I feel lives in "fear" of eating something wrong," says Tracey. "I want Kevin to have a healthy respect for his gluten intolerance, but I want him to know that he can *live* with Celiac. I want him to learn to make the right choices even though they may not be the fun choices. I want him to learn that even though he can't go out and eat pizza with his friends, he can go out with them and have a coke and salad."

Model Confidence

In other words, you want your child to feel he's just like everybody else, no matter what he eats—or doesn't eat. That means having enough of your own confidence and self-esteem to know how to handle a variety of situations in a variety of ways. If there's one area where it's particularly helpful to learn to think "outside the box", it's with food sensitivities.

Many families of food-sensitive children have evolved an entire culture of daily living that may sound daunting at first, but eventually leads to confident, comfortable children who can manage their own diets with a minimum of fuss and bother. Just keep reminding yourself that your role ends after a few years.

101

Ultimately, the dietary ball will be in your child's court, where it belongs. If you've done your part, though, his form should be great! Sometimes, it just takes a bit of chutzpah to confer that confidence to your child.

Think Outside the Box

"We typically pack our own food, and ignore signs saying 'no outside food', says Juliann. "You can ask for the ingredients at a restaurant during a slow time."

Karen even brings food from other restaurants. "Cody loves a double patty cheeseburger Happy Meal™ with

> *"I also have become very good at knowing what I can and can not eat. I read the labels and I know what is good and bad. You just have to get used to reading labels which is one thing almost nobody else does unless they like to stay healthy."—Jessica, 16*

no bun from McDonalds™. We have even taken his drive-through meal into the Chinese restaurant so the other kids could have the buffet they love. I talked to the managers before we did this and they said no problem. We get some funny looks coming in with Cody proudly carrying his McDonalds™ take-out box. But, oh well, he's happy!"

Sometimes she just brings food from home. "We have been to Pizza Hut™ with our own crust and they scrub out a pan, put on the toppings I request and bake our gluten-free pizza (for a small fee). We are then able to sit and eat with the wheat-eaters in the family that order in."

Role-Play Situations

☑ **As your child gets older, role-play situations that may come up in the course of a day; help your child feel comfortable avoiding temptation or peer pressure.**

Eventually, your child will be solely responsible for his or her diet. The earlier you begin educating your children about all the parameters of their health, the better. Children obviously can have a harder time eliciting and maintaining adult cooperation in their care than their parents will. The best thing you can do to ensure your child's safety when you're not there is to go to the extra effort of making sure all the parties involved know what is required of them. That also means making sure your child's caregivers know what the consequences are—in relation to your child's health and to their chances for continued employment— if the rules for your child's health are not followed to the letter.

The next thing you can do is to make sure your child knows what to do when things don't go the way they should. If adults insist your children eat something they know they shouldn't, be sure they know what recourses they have, either requesting assistance of another trusted adult—principal or daycare center manager—or calling home.

And certainly let them know that they can come to you without fear of blame if there have been problems in your absence. Try role-playing a variety of situations they might encounter during the day, and help them have ready answers to questions or polite refusals of foods in those situations. And teach your children to be firm in their explanations of their conditions as well.

Some stock replies that work well for us include:
- *"No, thank you."* This is usually Chris' first line of defense and often perfectly sufficient. It's simple, easy to say and understand, whatever a child's age, and it doesn't necessitate any more discussion. Only the most insistent relatives or strangers press him further.

- *"I can't have wheat (or milk, peanuts, corn, egg, or whatever the allergenic food)."* If pressed, this simple statement of exactly what can't be eaten sometimes does the trick. For some reason, people rarely question Chris when he says this. Maybe it's the strength of his conviction behind his words.

103

- *"I have a food allergy*." or *"I'm allergic to that."* That may not be completely accurate on a case-by-case basis, but it *is* something most people understand. Besides, "intolerance" is really hard to say when you're four.

- *"That makes me sick*." Aunt Edna might take offense at that remark, but it leaves nothing to the imagination. (It's better than "I'll throw up," which is a good response for follow-up questions, though.)

- *"I'll have to ask my mom (or Dad, or other responsible and aware adult)."* This is the answer of last resort, because you want your child to be able to deal with these situations himself as much as possible and you certainly don't want him to feel over-protected or look over-protected in front of other children. But your child should also know that, when pressed beyond endurance, it's perfectly acceptable to call in the reserves. Then you can do the explaining, and remind the insistent party that "No, thank you," means "No, thank you."

Nagging Concerns
Sometimes, there are those who simply don't want to accommodate others' special dietary (or other) needs. "How do we know that's really what's wrong?" Lee was asked. Others would say "Why should we have to care about what another child can eat—I don't want my child to feel deprived and who cares about some kid with problems."

The selfish, uncaring nature of such comments aside, these are serious, real-time concerns facing parents and children dealing with food sensitivities, issues that tend to rear their ugly heads at the most inopportune times. "I find that birthday parties and holiday get-togethers are the hardest to deal with when it comes to food allergies," says Cindy. "There are too many treats lying around during those times, and I usually find myself quite stressed by the end of the night."

Lindsay's poignant reflections express well the issues parents of food-sensitive children face both in the immediacy of the problem for their infants and toddlers, and their quite reasonable concerns for their children in the future.

"I can never relax at big parties—even though I put a sticker on Sam that says "Gluten Intolerant. Please don't feed me. "I still worry about him grabbing a cracker off the table. I used to worry about him finding gluten things on the floor and putting it in his mouth when he was younger but now it's off the table. I worry about people forgetting about his diet and handing him something along with the rest of the kids. Recently a friend and her baby were over to our home and the child dropped Cheerios™ all over the house as he toddled along— I was embarrassed to say something, angry I had to, and felt badly as I knew I was reacting unreasonably.

> "When I was younger I had a preschool teacher and we would have snacks right before nap-time. It would always be half of a certain fruit and a cup of milk. I would tell him that I couldn't drink the milk because my Mom told me not to and that I was allergic to it. He thought I was lying just to get out of drinking it and he would make me drink it anyway. When I would complain about stomach pains or needing to use the restroom during nap-time he was very unfeeling and I felt he was angry at me and I would become frustrated and angry."—Jane, 16

"I am angry when grandmothers send food gifts that I have to take away. I should be grateful as I realize he looks so "normal" they forget—and that is good in many ways. Most of all I worry about the future—his being the only child at Montessori not having the hot lunch, how as an adult he will fare at conventions and wedding reception banquets—things I should not worry about and spend my energy managing today so that he is knowledgeable and at ease enough to handle those things when they come up."

Make Your Child His Own Best Advocate

That, of course, is the key issue: helping our children become knowledgeable about their condition at an early age so they can handle things on their own later. No one understands or appreciates food sensitivities as well as those who have the sensitivity, so it's vital that your child, in the end, is his own best advocate.

Summing it All Up

- *Building a health advocacy team of caring family, friends, and caregivers* requires a threefold educational program: *Educate yourself...your child...and everyone around you!*

- *You can't leave anything to chance* when you're dealing with a food sensitivity, and you certainly can't abdicate your responsibility where your child's health is concerned. Here are some things you can do to keep family, friends, caregivers, and your food-sensitive child on the right track to good health:

  ☑ Make immediate family your child's primary support team.

  ☑ Before the school year begins, schedule meetings with teachers, school administrators, counselors, nurses, cafeteria personnel and office staff. Explain what foods cause a reaction, precautions, emergency procedures, how to read a label, and lunch time considerations. Have the same kind of meeting with family or friends who will be caring for your child. Be aware of your child's legal rights to a safe education.

  ☑ Make it as easy as possible for those on whose help you and your child rely to be able to provide that help.

  ☑ Keep and maintain a supply of snacks at your child's school or caregiver's or other family members' homes.

  ☑ Be involved in your child's daycare, school, or other activities.

  ☑ Empower your child by promoting healthy caution, not debilitating fear.

  ☑ As your child gets older, role-play situations that may occur; help him feel comfortable avoiding temptation or peer pressure.

  ☑ Develop an action plan for daycare, school, and work in the event of an allergic reaction: how to recognize reactions, medication needed (such as Benadryl or EpiPen), call 911, and call parents.

106

Chapter VI
Out in the World:
How To Help Your Child Fit In When He Can't Have His Cake and Eat It, Too

Once we got a handle on Chris' food sensitivity, and finished persuading, educating, and enlisting the help of family and friends in managing it—or at least accepting it, the next logical step was giving Chris as much control over his diet as was reasonably possible so he could go out and enjoy himself. Now admittedly, he's only seven, so he's not going out too far to enjoy himself.

But we do go to friends' homes, to birthday parties and picnics, on field trips and other outings, to restaurants, fairs and to family gatherings. I don't want to be hovering over him constantly, and I'm sure he'd rather not be hovered over constantly either. Since he's young and most of our friends, as well as the immediate family network of grandparents, aunts, uncles and cousins have literally grown up learning about his food intolerance with him, it hasn't been much of an issue in our usual social circle.

Chris amiably plucks carrot sticks and apples from fruit and vegetable trays, knows M&Ms™ are fine and, unless I've brought them, checks with me about the chips selections before going to town. And I usually bring an assortment of gluten-free treats anyway, so he never goes hungry.

When we're with a crowd of his peers, he holds his own pretty well, politely and confidently refusing offers of pretzels or cookies, explaining simply that he can't eat those foods because they make him ill. When pressed on just *how* those foods make him ill, he typically says something like "They make my stomach feel bad," or—the reply guaranteed to stop further questioning—"They make me go to the bathroom messy." He

107

also knows he can refer other parents and children to me for more information.

Chris and his Cousin

I remember one particularly touching scene at a restaurant outing with family. Chris was around four and his three-year-old cousin was trying quite insistently to share a muffin with him. "No thank you," Chris said. His cousin persisted. "Here. Eat dis!"

It took some effort, but I forced myself to stay out of it. Chris already knew his options in this situation. He could either say "Thank you" and simply put it aside and wipe his hands. Or, he could say, "No thank you," as he was trying to do with his cousin, and try to explain. I watched to see what he would do faced with such kind-hearted insistence.

He laughed. He told his cousin he couldn't eat wheat. His cousin frowned and shoved the muffin at him once more. Chris looked up at me, finally out of ideas. I explained gently to his cousin that Chris couldn't have wheat because it made him sick. "It makes you sick?" he asked. Chris nodded.

"Ohhhh," said his cousin with understanding. He returned to his mother at the other side of the table with the now mangled muffin in his fist. "He can't have the muffin," he explained to his mother. "It makes him sick."

Chris' cousin could identify with that. He'd been sick before and he didn't like it. Of course, not all children will be that easy to persuade or that sympathetic. But the more you let your child handle explanations, as well as his own choices of food, the better your chances are of producing a comfortable, happy child who controls his diet instead of allowing his diet to control him.

108

Building "Health-Esteem"

I'm fairly confident of Chris' ability to manage his diet well as he gets older. I've seen enough examples of his comfort levels in dealing with food issues, and his general gregariousness helps. He holds forth with complete ease on his dietary constraints with adults at church and in other settings where he's been offered forbidden food. On a couple of occasions, my heart skipped a beat when I realized I hadn't been nearby when the offending food was offered to him. But each time, he avoided problems with grace and charm.

At the other end of the spectrum, of course, are more naturally recalcitrant children who hate attention in any form. These are the children who, if they have a food sensitivity, suffer in silence, take abuse and teasing without seeking help, and are afraid to tell anyone about any physical discomfort they have. Or they hesitate to decline things for fear of being considered rude, or out of the greater fear of being pressed harder to have it anyway. These children require a little extra coaching and coaxing to learn to deal with their food sensitivities with the confidence necessary to carry them through a healthy life.

Sharon's Story

Sharon, for instance, has lived with food sensitivities all her life, and now deals with food sensitivities in her children, as well. She says she has spent her life apologizing for her illness and enduring foods she shouldn't eat because she's often simply too embarrassed to speak out.

"If you are at someone's house for a meal," Sharon laments, "sometimes they will have completely forgotten about our allergies and we end up with something one of us can't eat. "On one occasion, which was actually my sister-in-law's wedding, I knew they had been asked to provide for me. Also, I knew my mother-in-law had spoken to them and she knows exactly what I should eat. I told the waitress a gluten-free meal

109

is being provided for me and that my mother-in-law had asked for this. I waited while everyone else finished their starters.

"Then I was asked if soup would be suitable to me. I agreed and waited and waited. When it came it was gluten free because it was Heinz® Tomato soup and they apologized for it taking so long as someone had had to go out and buy it. Despite prior notice they seemed to have forgotten all about it. I was uncatered for in a good hotel where other people would have complained if they had received tinned soup." Sharon didn't complain, when complaint—or at least bringing the issue to the management's attention—was certainly warranted.

Typically, Sharon tries to phone ahead to restaurants she plans on eating in. "If you are speaking over the phone," she points out, "You are less likely to be embarrassed by having to be different on the night (of the restaurant outing). They may even, if they know in advance, offer to make you something suitable."

But when her outings don't work out as planned, if the catering fails or the wrong food is brought, she says, "I've just left when I'm ill or I don't want to be embarrassed. I do realize by not complaining someone else with a food intolerance will be ill but I spend so much of my life apologizing and being what they call awkward that I avoid this situation."

Sharon's story is an unhappy one sometimes. But we don't have to raise children who spend their lives apologizing for a medical condition, or who feel awkward in requesting perfectly ordinary things like "no bread." The sooner you start building your children's "health esteem," the sooner your children can be on the road to confident, healthy lives which *they* control.

Lorraine's Story
Lorraine has just such a family of children—nine of them to be exact—and all of them have celiac disease, as does Lorraine herself. It is more out of necessity than anything else that her

110

large family is as self-sufficient as possible in managing their own diets. And each of her children has personal reasons for staying or straying from their diets—as the case may be.

"Some of my children respond so violently to gluten that they *never* cheat," she says" because they will be vomiting and have diarrhea for three days." Although, she adds, that's "not to say they aren't tempted now and then by a good-lookin' donut." Her daughters have other reasons for sticking to a gluten-free diet. "My teen age girls let vanity rule because they become so bloated in their belly when they cheat. So they don't." (Well, they sometimes do "cheat," but it's rare and then it's also a conscious choice to do so.)

Although Lorraine home-schools her children and is able to provide most of their meals for them, her older daughter is in college now and dealing with her diet on her own. "Getting enough to eat at the college was difficult for her," she says. "She lived on dry salads and fruit unless she brought her own food from home which was difficult with her fast paced schedule and she lost quite a bit of weight this year. She's 5'7" and 108 lbs."

Nevertheless, she says, " My children are healthy now and we have adapted to this difficult lifestyle."

It's All in the Attitude
With something of a different perspective, Janet says," This is not a difficult thing to live with for us at all. We just incorporated it into our lives. We bought a tent-trailer for vacationing so that feeding Michael wouldn't be a problem and have become very outdoorsy," says Janet. "We volunteer for all the scouting week-ends to be cooks or leaders so we can have input on the meals to be provided.

"After all, the alternative is a sick (or worse) child. And anyone who saw how near a thing it was for Michael would not even consider cheating on the gluten-free diet. "

Whether you choose to look at it as adapting to a difficult lifestyle, or merely incorporating a new one, the point is it has to become *a* lifestyle. Obviously, the better your attitude about it, the better your child's attitude will be and the more seamlessly he or she can integrate into society at large. And there are lots of different ways to help your child adapt—or incorporate—his or her special diet into daily life with confidence and aplomb.

Be Creative!

"With a family as big as ours traveling is a feat anyway," says Lorraine. "We have found that camping is best because we can cook our own food over a campfire and we are all healthy. If I go somewhere in the van with them on the road, we stop at grocery stores instead of fast food chains so we can buy potato chips, string cheese, yogurt, sliced ham and cheese from the deli, and fresh fruit. This is "FAST FOOD" to us."

Start thinking outside the box and a whole new world of opportunity will open up for you and your children. For instance, suspend disbelief for a moment and entertain the possibility those perhaps "ordinary" cookies, candies, cake and breads are over-used and boring. Consider that vanilla or chocolate soy milk might be fun to share as class treats for a change.

Contribute exciting new things to your child's school snacks and treats[78]—like carrot sticks and hummus, or Chinese rice crackers (not the sweet American kind) or Jell-O™ jigglers or dried fruit or applesauce cups. Potato sticks are fun, too, and things like "ants on a log" (raisins on celery with cream cheese). Candies like M&M™s and Farley's™ or DelMontes™ fruit snacks are fun and safe for most kids, too.

---

[78] See the recipes in Chapter 11.

112

If your child knows from the very start that he has his own wide selection of special foods to choose from, chances are he'll not only choose them, but his enthusiasm will infect others who will enjoy eating his foods with him. My daughters routinely want to eat Chris' food, and love his special cookies as much as he does. And he's happy to share! You may have to remind your child, though, that although he can share his food with others, he should politely decline reciprocal sharing unless you or his (diet-educated) teacher gives him the okay.

Other foods that will make your child and his classroom contributions the envy of his classmates can include[79]:

Corn chips	Applesauce cups
Dried sweetened cranberries	Dried fruit[80]
	Fruit cups
Fried or dried vegetables such as peas, carrots	Mozzarella string cheese
	Nuts[81]
Gluten-free pretzels	Potato sticks
Jell-O™ jigglers	Prunes (dried plums)
Jell-O™ snack packs	Pumpkin seeds
M&M's™	Raisins
Popcorn	Sunflower seeds
Popcorn cakes	Trail mix
Popsicles	Yogurt
Potato chips	Homemade cake, cookies,
Pudding snack packs	bars, fudge, etc.

Janna's Story

When Janna's ten-year-old, gluten-intolerant daughter, Sara, was invited to join her Safety Patrol group on a trip to Washington D.C., the prospect initially provoked some anxiety in Janna. Then, with the support of gluten-free families on the Cel-Kids listserv[82], she got some creative suggestions and came up with a novel solution to the situation.

---

[79] Be careful about providing foods other children may be sensitive to or that may be inappropriate for certain ages, and edit this list according to your own child's sensitivities.

[80] If you're dealing with gluten intolerance, be aware that some dried fruit may be rolled in flour.

[81] Unless, of course, you're dealing with nut sensitivities!

[82] See Appendix for subscription information.

113

"I purchased two coolers: one large on wheels and one big enough for three meals. I packed each meal in individual plastic bags, labeled with which meal it was for. Each day, all she had to do was grab the three meals for that day and place them in her small cooler.

"Her teacher was responsible for keeping the large cooler filled with ice. It was cold in Washington...so keeping her smaller cooler fresh was not a problem. For breakfast I made waffles ahead of time that only had to be heated, hard-boiled eggs, yogurt, crisp rice bars, gluten-free cereal. Lunch was bologna, or ham, chips, Jell-O™, fruit, and cookies. Dinner was baked chicken or steak I made ahead of time, baked potatoes, veggies and anything left over from other meals from that day. I also packed snacks for her to choose from like microwave popcorn and brownies."

For the big trip "pizza party," Janna sent along a gluten-free pizza from Dietary Specialties™. "I arranged with the hotel to cook it for her. She did very well on her first trip away from home and had no accidental ingestions." Now *THAT'S* creative!

Let Your Child Be Responsible
As soon as you can, let your child be responsible for his or her diet. As with anything, if you show your children you trust them, generally your trust will be rewarded. And if you understand about occasional waywardness, they won't stray too often. Whenever possible, of course, stock them up with acceptable supplies, as Janna did. But understand that sometimes they're just going to have to choose for themselves from whatever is available. The better educated they are about their condition and their food choices, the more confident they will be and the less you'll have to worry.

Teach your child at an early age what foods are safe and what foods aren't. Make sure he knows how to keep his foods separate from foods that might cause problems at school, when you can't be with him. Even a young child can learn to use a napkin or a bandana as a place mat to keep his food from being contaminated by crumbs or residues on tables without much assistance. Your child can also eat right out of his lunchbox at school. Try to give him enough so he can share a little, but make sure he knows not to indulge in what others might want to share with him. The ability to share gives one confidence and helps build friendships.

"My kids have been attending church camps (and the like) all summer," says Lorraine. I have taken a cooler of "our" food with them. We include salad dressing (with no vinegar [83]), sour cream (with no mono & diglycerides), butter, gluten-free cookies, bread and muffins, and other stuff. The camps usually have fruit and salads available. However, my kids always come home a few pounds lighter. But at least they were without abdominal pain while they were there."

Jessica and Nicole
But otherwise, learn to trust them. Or at least, as they get older, give them room to learn to trust themselves. Two of Lorraine's daughters, Jessica and Nicole, make it plain that they decide what to eat and how diligently to stick to their diet, which they do *most* of the time.

Sixteen year old Jessica says," I usually can control my own diet myself. If I want to stay on my diet, I will. At home I eat wheat free most of the time because most of my family has this disease and my Dad, who doesn't, is on his own special diet anyway. So, most of the time I'm okay at home. It's when I get out and my mom isn't there telling me that I shouldn't eat this or that, even when she knows what it's like to crave what you can't eat. But that's when I eat whatever I feel like. Even when I know I'll regret it later."

---

[83] See Chapter 10 for a discussion on vinegar , which is now generally considered safe for celiacs and the wheat sensitive.

115

When she strays, Jessica has made a conscious decision to do so, despite the consequences. But nothing her mother could tell her at that point would make much of a difference. Jessica has reached a point where she is responsible; the results are up to her. On the other hand, Jessica also knows, "You feel so much better if you stay on your diet. You have energy and you feel almost normal."

Her twelve-year-old sister, Nicole, takes a more pragmatic approach to her situation." I just recently came home from …camp. In the cafeteria they had a variety of food that seemed so good. My mom had given me a box of cookies and cinnamon raisin bread (from the 'nutrition' section of our grocery store), a bag of homemade muffins, sour cream, and salad dressing. I didn't have very filling meals. I usually asked for an apple with my meager helpings of celiac food. But because I stuck with my diet I had a fantastic time, and most of the girls respected me for my will power."

That type of respect from peers is encouraging and inspiring for children. It puts them on top and in control. It makes them experts in their lives and leaders instead of followers. When others ask Nicole about her diet, she's happy to explain. "I usually tell them the grains I can't eat, name a couple of wheat by-products, what we use in wheat's place and if they ask, I tell them why we can't eat gluten."

Jane

Jane, 16, says her problem with milk has been somewhat alleviated as she's gotten older. But she knows who is responsible for her health. "Now that I'm much older milk doesn't affect me that much but if I do drink or eat something with an excess of milk I feel that it's harder for me to wake up and go to school. I sometimes feel like I'm bloated or have gastric problems that are very uncomfortable. It's really my decision to drink or eat milk products and I suffer the consequences on my own."

116

Use the Buddy System

It's also good for children to have a "buddy system" at school or in other peer situations. A "buddy system" can be older children who express an interest in helping a younger child, friends of food-sensitive child or older siblings. Your child's "buddies" should know what the symptoms of a food intolerance reaction look like, who to notify if they see one occurring and either what they can do to help or who they should alert.

Often "buddy systems" will occur naturally, and they're important to encourage. In our home, Chris' sisters form his buddy system. When he's playing with friends, they're usually familiar with his food sensitivity and often keep a look out for him. His best friend always checks with me before sharing food with him. "Can Chris have this?" she'll inquire earnestly each time. And all his "buddies" share enthusiastically in his treats.

He has to act fast among some non-food-sensitive friends to get his wheat-free brownies!

> *"Most of my friends are pretty understanding. MOST of them. I had a guy friend who lectured me for half an hour on how it was all in my head. He told me if I just eat it more my body will become immune to it."*—Jessica, 16

That leads to another consideration: We never tell his friends or anyone else that they can't have his food, even if it's expensive or difficult to make. The fact that others enjoy his food makes it seem more like well, just food, than anything that sets him apart from his friends. And the fact that Chris has something *he* can share with others is important and redeeming in itself.

Keep Things in Perspective

"We used to say that everyone has something wrong in their lives, " says Edith. "And there were worse things to have as problems than food sensitivities. Sometimes we would talk about what we were glad we didn't have to deal with, like being born with no legs or something. It kept things in perspective a little. "

Keeping a healthy perspective is paramount to keeping a healthy attitude about a food sensitivity and, indeed, about anything else. But especially where food is involved, it's important to stay levelheaded and not lose focus, or become overly self-absorbed. The last thing you or your children want to do is—pardon the pun—become consumed by food!

Some families maintain their perspective through their faith, others by keeping their eye on a silver lining and still others find comfort that their child's illness is something that can be controlled by diet alone. The most important thing to remember is that the better your perspective is, the better your child's will be.

> *"The best thing about [being a] celiac is you don't eat as much pre-prepared food or junk. Before we knew about the disease we would eat donuts for breakfast two to three times a week. And pizza three to four times a week. So you eat a lot more healthy in my opinion."*—Nicole, 12

"I don't think we should define the child by the diet as I feel many adult celiacs do," says Lindsay. "We all want our kids to be happy and well-adjusted; parents of celiacs just have more work to do in one area. One of my good friends told me that God never gives you more than you can handle. I am not particularly religious, but I thought of her perspective often this year."

"Be grateful for what you have—if these health problems can be solved by avoiding a few foods—thank goodness! Watching a friend whose child has cancer, and others whose children have other, more serious problems has taught me to count my blessings," says Lee.

> *"If I go somewhere and they serve me a dish that is really disgusting with an excess of milk in it that I don't want to eat, yet I don't want to be rude, I can use my allergy to excuse myself from eating that certain dish without being rude or feeling bad."*
> —Jane

"I think the most important thing I've

learned is that God gave Tyler celiac disease for a reason," says Danna. "In my case, I believe it was to help others through my Raising Our Celiac Kids (ROCK) group and book. There's always a reason."

The Silver Lining

Janet's silver lining is the over-all well-being of her entire family. "We all eat a lot of gluten-free food. For example, we all eat gluten-free cookies, muffins, pies, and cakes. I make gluten-free trail mix; we buy gluten-free hot dogs and spaghetti sauce. When I make pasta, I make two separate dishes and I make gluten-free bread only for Michael's consumption. Other than that we all eat basically the same things. We are SO healthy since none of us eat a lot of pre-packaged food."

> "Enjoy what you have because there are people who can't enjoy it the way you do."
> —Jessica, 16

Perhaps the most helpful perspective of all, though, is that—for the most part—it is, after all, just food we're dealing with; not respirators or ventilators, not dialysis machines, or blood transfusions. Food is something we and our children can manage.

"Most of all I feel grateful," says Lindsay. "I really thought Sam might die last year and to find out I 'only' have to manage his diet makes me feel lucky. But I also have a minor but nagging worry about him being 'alright'. I guess my advice is to raise the child to *live* with the diet restriction as a small part of their overall self."

Summing It All Up

- *Build "Health-Esteem"* in your child early.

- *Be creative* in your child's meals at home, the snacks he or she shares in school and what will be taken on special trips. The more varied, enjoyable, and inviting to others your child's food is, the more easily your child's diet will fit in with others.

119

- *Empower your child by* making your child responsible for his or her own meal and food choices as much as possible.

- *Use the buddy system,* by letting older children or your child's friends or siblings support him or her at school and elsewhere. This builds camaraderie and a sense of belonging.

- *Keep things in perspective* by reminding yourself that food sensitivities are usually problems that can be handled by diet alone and rarely require medical intervention. By keeping things in perspective, you can give your child a good attitude and "health-esteem" he can use for life.

Chapter VII
Eating Out:
"Burger... Hold the Bun, Please"

Learning to shop and cook gluten-free was a real confidence booster for us. After a while, we looked like chefs in the kitchen and professional buyers in the grocery store. Meals were a breeze, and shopping wheat free was second nature. We were in control of Chris' diet, and not controlled by it instead. We ran a tight food allergy ship and there was nothing a stray gliadin could do about it! But there was one thing, we discovered, that could take the wind out of the sails of our newly acquired health-esteem; something that had once been an occasion to celebrate, a culinary holiday, a family event:

EATING OUT!

At first, I viewed restaurants as something of an enemy, a shape shifting, ambiguous adversary defined by things I couldn't see, taste, or smell but somehow threw my son's gut into disarray if I failed to be vigilant. When Chris was very young, my greatest source of consternation was the number of breaded foods on children's menus. We rarely ate at fast food restaurants, which actually tend to be fairly reliable places as far as food sensitivities go (but less as far as fat, cholesterol, and nutrition go!).

But it seemed like everything suitable for a child was dredged in flour! Everywhere I looked, I saw bread. It was like when I became pregnant and suddenly there were pregnant women everywhere. Now everywhere I looked, I saw wheat.

Restaurants, especially, seemed to run white with flour. Yeast rolls and little loaves of rye or wheat before meals, croutons in the salad, breaded mozzarella sticks for appetizers, flour based seasonings for chicken, fish and meat, giant breaded blooming onions, crackers in the soup, flour based gravy on the potatoes,

121

and big, thick, doughy pizza crusts. What, you may well ask (as I did), is the dining out family of a food-sensitive child to do?

Adapt and Learn

First, get over it. My first response to eating out with Chris was a mild sense of panic. Then I realized that it was just a matter of thinking outside the box again. Restaurants have trained us to feed our children off the children's menu when that's hardly a requirement for eating out. As a matter of fact, I quite agree with those who have been calling for simply scaled-down versions of adult meals for children, rather than the limited, often less healthy, selections frequently offered. We learned how to order meals for our son differently, and you can too.

Second, learn to negotiate the restaurant maze with the same agility as the grocery store/labeling maze. That means learn which restaurants carry the greatest variety of foods your child can enjoy. Find out which are the most "Allergy Aware" (more on this Canadian concept later), and which are the most open to working with diners with special needs—and there are many restaurants out there now that are willing to do so. Learn how to dine out by calling ahead, researching menus and maximizing your outing by bringing along your own "appetizers" to get your child through the waiting period for the entrée.

Dining out is a major hurdle for many families, and all develop their own special ways of doing it—which sometimes means not doing it.

"We rarely go out to eat," says Tracey. "That used to be a "social" activity for the family. We used to go out at least three to four times a month."

"We can't be spontaneous and eat new foods for fun," laments Juliann. So they compromise. " We typically pack our own food, and ignore signs saying 'no outside food'."

122

"I know we are taking risks eating in restaurants," admits Lindsay. "And I do my best to minimize the risks. [I look for] hamburger cooked in a clean pan, eggs in a clean pan, baked potatoes, fruit. I can find something in almost any restaurant but a pizza or pasta place."

"Going out to eat is the greatest challenge." Lynda agrees. " At home it is no big deal. We pretty much all eat gluten free except for bread and pasta. But we just got back from our trip to Orlando—[it was] pretty frustrating. [We were] always thinking about what Nathan would be able to eat. I bring his own bread and buns when we go out and a few snacks. Nathan isn't a great eater so we are also dealing with that."

"We plan eating out," says Barbara. "It is seldom spontaneous. We have 'planned reactions', allowing foods that are not normally eaten for some specific reason. When we have a 'planned reaction', we are ready and our patience is at a much higher level."

But most families find a way to continue eating out together. And realistically, it's a good idea to do so at least occasionally. If your goal is to normalize your child's life as much as possible, that's going to have to include eating away from home. Like everything else, the key to eating out successfully is to educate yourself about the restaurants you plan to patronize. Fortunately, restaurants are starting to educate themselves about food sensitivities, too.

Restaurants Sit Up and Take Notice

In Canada, there has been a strong movement by the Canadian Restaurant Association, in conjunction with local allergy associations, to better educate restaurateurs about allergies. Restaurants that show a measure of understanding and a willingness to assist diners on special diets display an "Allergy Aware" sign outside their facilities, to let food-sensitive diners know they can (hopefully) eat safely at that establishment.

123

European food associations have also responded positively to increasing incidents of severe allergic reactions to food. There, the Anaphylaxis Campaign, along with the Ministry of Agriculture, Fisheries and Food, and representatives of the British food industry have created guidelines for providing customer information to diners and catering customers.[84]

Managers of food service industries are encouraged to be well-educated regarding food sensitivities and to always have at least one staff member on hand who is well versed in the various ingredients of the foods and recipes used at the facility.

They're urged to use special precautions in kitchens and serving areas to minimize cross-contamination problems, and to note on menus where nuts or other allergens may be an issue so that customers can make safe dining choices. Customers are even encouraged to question staff and the Anaphylaxis Campaign suggests signs be displayed stating, "We welcome inquiries from customers who wish to know whether any meals contain particular ingredients."

On the Home Front

It's not likely you'll find a sign like that in too many U.S. restaurants. But even here, food sensitivities are gaining recognition as the serious issue that they truly are. In November 1999, the State of Maryland created a Task Force on Food Allergies and Restaurant Patrons (Chapter 226, Acts of 1999). The Task Force was charged with examining the concerns of, and problems encountered by food-sensitive diners. The Task Force plans to consult with the federal Food and Drug Administration about food labeling laws and policies, and to address problems and concerns and possible resolutions to these issues by April 30, 2001.

---

[84] Anaphylaxis Campaign, 2 Clockhouse Road, Farnborough, Hampshire GU14 7QY. Write Admail 6000, London SW1A 2XX for more information. Please quote Ref PB3317 (for poster), PB3318 (for booklet), and PB3406 and PB3407 (for stickers). Telephone 0645 556000.

In addition, The National Restaurant Association is now working with the Food Allergy Network and the American Academy of Allergy, Asthma, and Immunology to better educate restaurant owners and staff nationwide. The three organizations recently produced and distributed 30,000 pamphlets about food allergies to association members. The pamphlets, *"What You Need to Know About Food Allergies,"* discuss different types of food sensitivities, how restaurants can help food-sensitive customers, and advises them on how to deal with food reactions.[85]

They also created a poster called "Understanding Food Allergy," designed to "give employees a basic understanding of food allergies."[86] The poster illustrates food that may cause sensitivities, lists symptoms of food sensitivities, and provides suggestions for treating food sensitivities in restaurant settings.

The point is, saying "My child is sensitive to wheat," or to peanuts or eggs or soy or corn or milk shouldn't bring the restaurant roof caving in anymore, especially if you call ahead and discuss this with the restaurant management in advance.

Calling Ahead
As with almost every issue in food sensitivities, good communication skills go a long way towards enhanced health and safety. Just as you have to make sure your child's caregivers and teachers are educated about your child's condition, so you have to communicate your needs to the restaurant you're visiting or plan to visit. We're talking here, of course, about traditional sit-down, multi-course meal service rather than fast food sizzle and serve; perhaps the type of place you'd take the family after church or for get-togethers with friends or relatives for special occasions or holidays.

---

[85] From "Food allergies, rare but risky," FDA Consumer Magazine.
[86] The National Restaurant Association, 1200 Seventeenth St., NW, Washington, D.C., 202.331.5900, e-mail: info@dineout.org

At one particularly fine restaurant where we joined family for a large celebration, we explained Chris' problem to the maitre d' when we arrived and he sent the chef over to talk to us after we were seated. After a short discussion, he decided to create a scaled down version of one of their broiled steak dinners, without the sauce typically served there, and with steamed vegetables and potatoes for Chris. It was a great dinner, and a number of us looked longingly at it as we ate our own, which tended to be fancy sauce covered things with seasoned vegetables. Chris' definitely looked much tastier!

Keep It Simple and Clear
Generally, though, at whatever restaurant you dine, your best bet is to select minimally prepared foods from the adult menu for your child. Even if the restaurant won't pare down the price accordingly, it's just safer for your child to have grilled or broiled meats and lightly cooked vegetables (providing the chef knows the cooking area must be free of contaminants).

Sometimes you can just order such a meal for yourself and split it with your child, which we've done on several occasions. In nearly four years, across several states, in a variety of restaurants, we've never had anyone complain when we ask to share meals with Chris, or if we need a smaller version of an adult meal. Communicating clearly and honestly with restaurant staff goes a long way towards comfortable, happy dining for all.

When you call to make a reservation be sure to mention your child's food sensitivity. Remind the staff when you arrive that you have a food-sensitive diner with you, and explain clearly what your child can and cannot eat. Most good restaurants are willing to go to reasonable lengths to make their diners comfortable, and they don't want diners to suffer discomfort during their visit. So don't be afraid to talk to people.

About the only thing really lost as you learn the ropes of dining out, is a sense of spontaneity, and even that can be regained, to

126

some extent, with experience. As a matter of fact, with a little foresight and planning, you'll soon find you can eat out with reasonably relaxed confidence—exactly the type of behavior you want to model for your child. You just have to keep in mind that relaxed confidence can't come without that foresight and planning.

Dining Out Safely

If you explain your situation to restaurant owners and staff, they're usually willing to overlook the oddities of dining out with food sensitivity. That means they'll turn their heads the other way when you walk into an Italian restaurant with a gluten-free Happy Meal for your child, or ignore the Tupperware containers of special food next to the Blooming Onion.

Food Allergy Survivors Together (FAST) offers some good tricks and tips to make your dining out experience as pleasant as possible. Here are a few of their suggestions, combined with some others I've picked up along the way:

✂ *Avoid high-risk restaurants* where items your food-sensitive child can't eat are likely to be served with some frequency. Even if you order something "safe", the dangers of cross contamination are considerably higher in these types of restaurants. Celiacs, the peanut-allergic, and soy-allergic should avoid Asian restaurants where peanut oil, soy, and wheat are used a lot. Italian restaurants can be tough on the gluten-intolerant. Mexican restaurants aren't a good idea if your child is sensitive to corn.

✂ *Eat at restaurants that already cater to special diets*—like kosher, vegetarian, or health food restaurants.

✂ *Eat at hotels, fine restaurants, or small restaurants*. All three are usually more accommodating than fast food restaurants or chains. And frequent staff turnover at better restaurants is less of an issue than at chains, where it's difficult to establish rapport.

✗ ***On the other hand, many chains are now responding to customer demand*** and you can often get a list of foods that are gluten-free, casein-free, etc. from the more popular chain restaurants.

✗ Restaurants like Burger King™ and McDonalds™ now offer ingredient lists and identify where cross-contamination can occur. Tony Roma's™ also has a reputation for being friendly to the food-sensitive. One FAST member reported that at one Tony Roma's™, the staff brings labels out to diners or invites them into the kitchen. They even have different grills for different meats. (See the next section for getting ingredient information from chain restaurants.)

✗ ***When you find a "safe" restaurant, patronize it with some regularity*** so the staff (better yet, the chef) gets to know you and your family. If you can, let them know what ingredients are best for you. Make friends with the staff and learn all about their cooking techniques and routine. Casual conversation will reveal the types of oils used in cooking, or whether flour is dusted on different foods like potatoes or other vegetables.

✗ ***Key questions to ask***, of both regular and fast food restaurants should include things like:

✗ "Are hamburgers all beef with no fillers?"

✗ "Is flour used for seasoning or dusting French fries or any other foods?" If so, ask what types of flours are used.

✗ "Are foods like French fries or sweet potato chips cooked in "clean" oils, and not contaminated by recycled oils used for things like fried, breaded chicken or onion rings or fish?"

✗ "Do you use soy in any way (if soy is a problem)?

✕ "What type of oils do you use? Peanut, canola, or something else?"

✕ "Are grilled meats or poultry marinated in anything and are the marinades shared by beef, chicken, fish, etc.?"

✕ "Is the grill cleaned between uses, or are separate grills used for different types of foods?"

✕ *When you contact restaurants to discuss your child's food sensitivities prior to a visit, call early in the day*, before they get busy. Explain your child's situation and ask for recommendations from the manager or staff. Find out if the restaurant prepares its meals from scratch or uses pre-packaged ingredients. Scratch is safer and more reliable.

✕ *Request sauces, condiments, and dressings on the side* to avoid cross-contamination or allergens, or bring your own.

✕ *Carry safe foods with you everywhere*. Emergency bananas, apples, and other safe snack foods are lifesavers, especially if service is slow. A small, soft-sided cooler with safe snacks like fruit leather, rice cakes, chips, dried fruit, or cut-up veggies in a baggie can go a long way towards making your restaurant visit an enjoyable one for everyone.

✕ *Keep a list of your child's food sensitivities with you at all times*, along with a list of acceptable foods that your child can eat, and a note about the dangers of cross-contamination. This helps you order, and also provides restaurant staff with a little hands-on education.

✕ *Always carry needed medications when you're out*. If your child depends on epinephrine during a reaction, you need to make sure it's always within reach. Carry antihista-mines such as Benadryl, as well. Make sure fellow diners are aware of the problem and know what to do if your child has a reaction and you've stepped away briefly.

✕ *Consider joining a dining club* [87] if you and your family travel and eat out a lot.

The Value of Menu and Ingredient Lists

Getting menu and ingredient lists from restaurants has never been easier. Most chain restaurants have websites, often with their menus and nutritional information available right online. Some places, like McDonald's™, even go the extra step to break their menu down by food allergen for their diners. You can call or write any restaurant and ask for specific menu information and usually you'll get it. If you're not convinced the information you're hearing is accurate, of course, then go with your instincts and dine elsewhere. But for the most part, good restaurants are happy to provide you with menu information.

The Helpful...

Writing to Taco Bell™[88], for instance, will get you an answer like this: "Because wheat is a part of so many of our recipes, many items served in Taco Bell™ restaurants are not suitable for gluten-restricted diets. However, there are a few items you can safely order:

Pintos and Cheese	Nachos Bellgrande (no beef)
Bean tostada	Cheese sauce
Nachos	Guacamole
Nachos supreme (no beef)[89]	Hot or mild sauce

Burger King's™ (BK) list of ingredients helps alert diners to more than meets the eye. As per BK's website, one BK Broiler™—ostensibly just a broiled chicken breast—contains, in addition to the chicken: water, seasoning (salt, chicken stock, flavoring, maltodextrin, and autolyzed yeast), partially hydrogenated soybean oil, and sodium phosphates.

---

[87] See Appendix.

[88] Please contact all restaurants of interest for the most recent information, as ingredient lists and recipes change over time.

[89] Taco Bell™ uses a beef extender and doesn't recommend it for the gluten free diet.

130

And it's glazed with: water, seasoning (maltodextrin, salt, chicken stock, hydrolyzed soy protein, flavors) modified food starch, methylcellulose gum, monosodium glutamate, soy sauce (wheat, soybeans, salt) chicken fat, hydrolyzed wheat gluten, xanthan gum, natural smoke flavor, partially hydrogenated soybean oil, butter (cream, salt) hydrolyzed corn gluten, auto-lyzed yeast extract, buttermilk, corn syrup solids, thiamine hydrochloride, citric acid, lactic acid, caramel color, disodium inosinate, disodium guanylate, vegetable stock (carrot, onion, celery, paprika, and tocopherol) and partially hydrogenated soybean oil."

Similarly, their French fries consist of "potatoes and partially hydrogenated vegetable shortening (soybean oil), modified potato and cornstarch, rice flour, dextrin, salt, leavening (sodium acid pyrophosphate, sodium bicarbonate), corn syrup solids, xanthan gum, and dextrose."

But Burger King™ has provided a wonderful service by disclos-ing ingredients so thoroughly. Because I also know that their burgers are really 100% beef (no fillers), my son can eat a bur-ger (no bun), while I indulge in the BK Broiler™ if I so choose.

Denny's™ will provide a list of menu items that might be "of concern to people diagnosed with the condition of Celiac Sprue" (and no doubt with other conditions as well). But it also warns that "this listing is based on authorized products and vendors" and consumers "may want to verify the absence of avoided ingredients in products by looking at the actual product labels of suspect items you are considering to choose. In addition, we may change vendors or reformulate products."

These are excellent points and Denny's™ is wise to make them. It encourages consumers inquiring about their food items to "check back with us routinely for an updated listing," which is good advice when checking into any restaurant items anywhere.

131

Wendy's™ includes "Other Gluten-Related Information" on their gluten-free lists, which is quite helpful and reassuring. About their cheese sauce, the information sheet says, "The hydrolyzed vegetable protein in the cheese sauce is derived from corn and soybean." The natural flavoring in their chili is "soluble spices including white pepper, clove, allspice, and cinnamon." All modified food starch in Wendy's™ food, advises the sheet, "is derived from corn." Their grilled chicken, they explain, "does not contain any flour or gluten-based ingredients. Flavorings and colorings (caramel) are all corn based. The maltodextrin is derived from corn." Wendy's™ also warns, "due to the daily rotation of oil in our fryers, there is a chance that the fries could be cooked in oil previously used to cook breaded chicken nuggets or fish."

This is all tremendously helpful information, and I, for one, feel reassured ordering in a restaurant where I'm able to get such precise ingredient information.

...And the Not-So-Helpful
And then some restaurants are a little less accommodating. One well-known restaurant addresses inquiries about its menu items thusly: "Because (our) menu is large and the combinations numerous, it is not feasible to produce a brochure of nutritional facts as some of our fast food colleagues have done."

They do point out that they have "been addressing the issue of fats, sodium, and cholesterol by introducing alternative items on our menu" and that they also have "many healthy alternatives within the parameters of our concept." Those, the restaurant says, include entrée salads, turkey sausage, and grilled chicken and fish. That said, one would still have to ask specific quest-ions about what's in the turkey sausage and wonder if the grilled chicken and fish is contaminant-free.

Individual restaurants vary as to the extent of their cooperative-ness, but that's what you base your dining loyalty on anyway. A restaurant's response to your inquiries will tell you as much as anything else about your child's safety there.

Stay on Top of Things

Two things are important here: One, unless you find particularly cooperative restaurant management at a small local restaurant or at a chain franchise, the best way to get relevant menu information is to call or write the main office of a restaurant. And two, you can't rest on your laurels once you've accrued a file folder of restaurant data. As always, your diligence is paramount to your child's health, and you should check back regularly with the restaurants you frequent to see what, if anything, has changed in their menus.

What to Ask and Whom to Ask

If you eat out a lot, or simply have a favorite restaurant or two that you'd like to continue dining at with your family, despite your child's food allergies, talk to the management first. If you're satisfied with their suggested menu items or lists of ingredients, then you're all set to go. If you'd rather have more precise information from a chain-type restaurant like Applebee's™ or the Boston Cooker™, then you need to contact that restaurant's main headquarters with your inquiries.

In most cases, you'll want to contact a company's consumer services office or department. Be very specific in your letter about what you want to know. Don't ramble. Nobody needs to know you or your child's entire history. The more concise your letter of inquiry is, the more precise the response can be.

A simple and polite letter like the following will do nicely.

> *Dear Sir or Madam,*
>
> *"I enjoy dining in your restaurant, but my child has a food sensitivity and we need to be careful diners. My child has celiac disease, which means he must avoid "gluten" containing foods such as wheat, barley, oats, and rye. Could you provide me with a list of your gluten-free foods, please, if one is available? Otherwise, a list of the ingredients you use in your main menu items (or children's menu items), including preservatives or additives, would be just as helpful.*
>
> *"Thank you very much."*

If your child is lactose intolerant, briefly list the foods your child cannot eat. You don't have to list everything, just the foods you feel would be most likely to occur in a restaurant setting. Ask about specific menu items you order regularly. Use the same format if your child cannot consume casein proteins, peanuts, corn, soy or eggs. You might want to enclose a "fact sheet" about your child's food sensitivity, there are examples printed in the back of this book.

Sometimes when you're dining out and don't have the benefit of a restaurant list with you, it's helpful for the waitstaff and the chef if you can list the things your child *can* eat safely in the restaurant. For instance, when we're dining out, I always tell the staff that my son can't eat wheat, but then explain that grilled meats or poultry prepared on clean surfaces are fine, as well as baked potatoes with condiments on the side, or steamed or lightly cooked vegetables. If your child can't eat corn, then suggest corn-free meals the restaurant might be able to provide. It helps the staff get in the right frame of mind, and takes some of the burden off of them for making the right decision for you.

Remember, the more aware we make restaurants about food sensitivities, the more likely they will be considerate of food-sensitive diners, and the more conscious they will be of the ingredients they use in their foods.

Again, the idea shouldn't be to make unfair demands upon restaurants, any more than upon food manufacturers. But educated restaurants are more likely to be safe ones, simply because they don't want to lose customers and will find ways to make their more popular foods safe for as many people as possible.

Summing it All Up

- *Learn to think outside the box* **when it comes to eating out. Order "safe" foods for your child from the adult menu, if none are available on the children's menu. And use your food sensitivity savvy to help your child dine out safely anywhere you go.**

- *Some safe dining tips include:*
  - *Avoid high-risk restaurants* **such as Asian places if your child is gluten intolerant or soy sensitive, or Mexican restaurants if your child is sensitive to corn.**
  - *Become familiar with safe restaurants* **by talking to managers and chefs, and reward those restaurants with your patronage, and be aware of restaurant staff turn-over as a factor in safety.**
  - *Call ahead whenever possible,* **to let the restaurant know you will have a food-sensitive diner with you and to discuss safe menu items beforehand.**
  - *Know what questions to ask,* **including questions about cross contamination risks, types of oils used in cooking, types of seasoning used, and kitchen habits.**
  - *Request condiments and sauces on the side.*
  - *Keep a list of your child's food sensitivities with you,* **along with a list of safe foods for ordering reminders.**

- *Always take safe foods with you* for your child to munch on while awaiting the main course, or in the event that a meal is unsuitable.
- *Always keep your child's medications with you,* especially if there is a danger of anaphylactic shock.
- *Consider joining a special diets dining club,* if you eat out frequently.
- *The more you know about a restaurant's menu ingredients, the more safely you can dine. Request menu ingredients online, by phone, or with a letter.*

- *Restaurants vary in degree of cooperativeness, but most will reply to a polite letter which should include:*
  - *A brief description of your child's food sensitivity.*
  - *Possibly a fact sheet describing it in better detail, with brief lists of permissible and forbidden foods.*
  - *And a request for the restaurant's "safe" foods for your child, or a list of the ingredients they use in their menu items.*
- *Help the waitstaff and the chef help you by making suggestions of what your child CAN eat in their restaurant.*

- *The idea is not to make unfair demands of restaurants, but to educate them about food sensitivities to make dining safer for more people.*

Part III
Eat, Drink, and Be Merry:
Cooking for Health and Happiness

Chapter VIII
Menu Planning:
How to Feed Everyone Without Cooking Twice

While dining out gives most families a break, dining out for families with food-sensitive members can be something of a chore. Sure it's fun, once you get the hang of it. But with all the preparations that go into going out, it often seems like less work just to stay home and cook! At least if you make it yourself, there's no doubt in your mind—or your child's—about what's in the food.

And there are a few other perks, too. Eating at home enjoying meals you fix yourself enriches your family life, restores some very basic, fundamental living skills to your life, and improves everyone's health and well-being. As a matter of fact, learning to cook for your food-sensitive child can very well turn out to be one of the best things that could happen to you and your whole family.

One Family, One Meal
Since we discovered Chris' problem when he was very young, we could integrate his wheat-free meals with our "regular" ones without much trouble. I didn't see any benefit to fixing special meals for him and other meals for the rest of the family. That would just mean a lot of time in the kitchen for me, and less time with my young family who often needed me elsewhere.

Typically, I fix a main entrée and then a selection of side dishes, such as rice and beans or baked potatoes and a couple of different plates of steamed or lightly cooked vegetables from which to choose. So, if we were having breaded baked chicken, for instance, I simply substitute corn meal or potato chips for the bread coating and prepare a single baked chicken dish.

Instead of rolls or muffins with meals, we eat corn bread or corn chips. We have Jell-O™ instead of cookies or cake for dessert, or our special wheat-free fudge for a treat. The end result has been that Chris, from an early age, learned to eat the same things as everyone else and everyone else, more or less, eats the same things he does. And I don't spend all my time cooking.

On picnics or other outings, we simply take along a big selection of goodies that both he and his sisters enjoy— everything from granola bars for the girls to wheat-free trail mix for Chris, and lots of fruit for everybody. If we go to a restaurant, I always make sure I bring "appetizers" Chris enjoys so he can have something he likes while we munch on yeast rolls waiting for our meal. Almost from the start, eating wheat-free became routine for us. And many families have found the same thing to be true for them.

A Non-Issue
"It's a non-issue in our home," says Danna. "I feel strongly that we should not make it a big deal. He is the only one completely gluten-free (we eat "regular" pasta and bread, for instance), but most of our meals tend to be gluten free just because it's easier on me that way. We eat gluten-free salad dressings, spaghetti sauces (add sauce later to cooked pasta), and so on."

Lindsay's experiences are similar. "In our home, gluten free has become a non-event," she says. "We have adapted, are aware of cross-contamination, and just quit eating pasta and yummy gluten desserts. I put my energies into gluten-free recipes."

Of course, if you're dealing with multiple food allergies in the family, or if children have different food allergies, you're going to have to adapt a bit differently. But with good menu planning and providing a variety of easy to fix selections with meals, feeding your food sensitive child or children shouldn't really entail a lot more work for you.

"It's funny, but we never ate all that much 'forbidden' food to begin with," says Lee. "We have always eaten a lot of rice and potatoes, and veggies—my oldest is allergic to virtually all preservatives and artificial additives, so that has been much more of a challenge! Main meals are almost unchanged—treats and home baked goods have been the only items that have become a challenge."

The general consensus seems to be that if you always cooked regular family meals from scratch from the beginning, going gluten free or dairy free or avoiding other allergens isn't that big of a deal. If, on the other hand, you're a self-described "McDonald's Queen" like Lorraine, *then* you've got a little adjusting to do.

"This diet hasn't been easy for me," says Lorraine," as I believe I was 'McDonald's Queen' before we found out about this disease five years ago." Now, she says, "I grind my own short grain brown rice into flour and special order 25 lb. bags of tapioca flour to make my own bread. I also grind popcorn into flour for corn bread. I make my own mayonnaise and salad dressings and make a lot of soups."

What's Available?
With the exploding popularity of health foods, you don't even have to do that unless you really enjoy grinding grains yourself. You can buy potato flour, tapioca flour, bean flours, soy flour and more, without too much fear of cross-contamination if you're buying from the more reliable mills. You can pick up gluten-free and other "allergen-free" cereals in some of the mainstream grocery stores' health food sections, now, too, along with gluten-free and dairy-free snacks, cookies, and cakes, if you're really devoted to convenience snack foods. Prepared wheat-free baking mixes for pancakes, waffles, and

139

muffins are excellent. And, there are several lines of boxed rice or other grain mixes from which you can prepare rather exotic but allergen-free meals for a minimum of money and time.[90]

"We all eat a lot of gluten-free food," says Janet. "For example, we all eat gluten-free cookies, muffins, pies, cakes. I make gluten-free trail mix; we buy gluten-free hot dogs, spaghetti sauce, etc. When I make pasta, I make two separate dishes and I make gluten-free bread only for Michael's consumption. Other than that we all eat basically the same things."

Mixing It Up

The biggest problem we've encountered, which is more of a nuisance issue than a true "problem" (if we're keeping things in perspective!), is keeping our meals varied enough to be interesting. It's easy to fall into the somewhat dull routine of meats and chicken and the same vegetables simply because, well, they're easy to fix. Most families alleviate that problem by ordering pizza once a week or going out for burritos or to an Italian restaurant. Those aren't really options for the gluten-free or dairy-free family, and that's where a little more planning and creativity come in.

The secret here—which isn't really much of a secret—is good menu planning. Plan ahead a little and you can keep meals interesting and still limit the amount of work it takes to create a good meal. Good menu planning also makes rotation diets possible, which is another way to alleviate food sensitivity issues.

Menu planning is also a nice, positive experience, since it focuses exclusively on what you and your family *can* eat and not on what you *can't* eat. If you have your meals planned out for a week or two, with healthy, varied food selections shining out at you from your completed menu plans tacked on the fridge, you and your food-sensitive children are less likely to

---

[90] See Vendors in Appendix.

have that sinking "There's nothing to eat" feeling. And that's a pretty dismal feeling when there really IS nothing safe to eat!

Menu Planning, Step 1: Explore Your Options

This is a fun step. After you figure out what your child can't have, go out with your "okay" list (see Chapter 9) and have at it! Take your food-sensitive child shopping and—together— find all sorts of appropriate foods to try. Go ahead and buy stuff and try stuff you've never bought or tried before.

Try some new alternative grains, make up gluten-free baking mixes, invest in a bread machine, and try out some gluten-free breads. Try a pre-made, wheat-free baking mix and make some of the recipes on the bag's side. Get rice flour and make pancakes. Check out the non-dairy butters, soy milk, egg replacers, and almond butter. Don't worry about making your foods match right now. This is your experimental period. Go for it!

Spend some time getting to know your child's diet as a family. You might be surprised to find that some of the new foods are really tasty and satisfying. Think ethnic, if possible, and try Mediterranean and Middle Eastern dishes. Go Asian; use wheat-free tamari sauce if wheat's the problem. Try stir-fry cooking with safe oils. Make rice pilafs, fruit salads, or bean salads.

Expand Your Horizons

One healthy diet that doesn't get much press but makes a lot of sense from a low food toxicity perspective is the "Paleolithic Diet,"[91] or what I like to call the "Early Man" diet. It consists largely of fresh fruit and vegetables, lean meat, poultry, fish, nuts, and small amounts of eggs and olive oil.

Of course, you'd have to remove those aspects of the diet to which your child is sensitive, but the basic premise is the same

---

[91]From PaleoFoods, with permission by Don Wiss. See a collection of discussions on this diet at the Paleolithic Diet Page, http://www.paleodiet.com

141

one I've always used in our meals: plain, pure, simple foods are the healthiest.

Typically, those on the Early Man diet eat when they're hungry, and never worry about calories or fat. The diet relies on a variety of foods chosen on the basis of whether they *could* be eaten raw. This includes meat and fish, which are only cooked because of bacteria concerns but which could be—and in some parts of the world are—eaten and digested in their raw forms. A meal might consist of trail mix and fresh fruit, or lean steak or chicken with cooked vegetables and a salad.

The point is, despite the shock you may experience when you discover all the things your food-sensitive child *can't* eat, there is a great deal he or she

> *"It might sound disgusting, but (I like) green apples with peanut butter. Another thing (I like) is apple pie. I like rice. I like hot dogs (Oscar Mayer™). I like waffles, when mom makes them. She uses applesauce instead of milk in the recipe."*—Miri, 7

still *can* eat. It's just a matter of changing paradigms. Expand your culinary horizons! Try everything with enthusiasm, no matter what you think of the taste. And don't make any faces!

I've often found that dishes that don't appeal to me are my son's favorites. But if I even suggest that I may not like something then he may decide not to eat it, too. Right now, you must be a dietary role model by not influencing your child with your own prejudices. Let your child decide—with encouragement toward the varied and healthy—what he likes, then go with those preferences.

Substitutes Galore!

Here are a few "rules of thumb" to get you started. Then use the recipes, tables, and lists in subsequent chapters to find appropriate foods that you can mix and match, or with which to create your own recipes.

First of all, become familiar with food families. Food families are the master lists of things like mustards, legumes, grains and parsley. If you've been told your child is sensitive to "legumes" for instance, that means you have to avoid things like peas, peanuts, and limas. (See Food Families in Appendix.)

Second, learn what substitutions[92] are available and how to use them to replace your forbidden ingredient(s). As noted earlier, it's usually wheat, dairy, and eggs that need replacing so here's a quick overview.

> "*My (favorite) meal would have to be mashed potatoes, the real potatoes that come out of the ground, with milk and butter in them. And corn, roast beef and gravy. The gravy is made with cornstarch, milk and the meat juice after it's cooked. My snack would have to be cheese melted onto corn chips. My treat would have to be the recipe we have for gluten free chocolate chip cookies. The best ever. I could make those every day!*"—Jessica, 16

Typically, in place of wheat flour we use a flour mix[93], blended from different combinations and proportions of flours made of rice, beans, corn, potatoes, sorghum, tapioca, arrowroot, soy, and so on. Different flours and flour mixes produce different textures and flavors. Xanthan gum—or guar gum—must be used to prevent crumbling in baked goods. Cooking times may vary and there are a few new techniques, but basically it's cooking from scratch.

Dairy products, especially milk, are easily replaced by beverages made from rice, soy, almonds, oats (unless you're gluten-sensitive), and potatoes—or 3/4 as much water or juice. Be sure

---

[92] Look at Chapter 10 for more complete substitution information.
[93] See Chapters 10 and 11.

143

to read labels to avoid other allergenic ingredients in so-called dairy-free items. Some "dairy-free" cheeses contain casein (milk protein).

Replacing eggs is a little more challenging, especially in baking where they play an integral role—and especially if you're baking with gluten-free flours. But very satisfactory results are possible using substitutes such as soft silken tofu or flaxseed meal or pureed fruit such as bananas or applesauce.

Menu Planning, Step II

Once you get yourself accustomed to substitutions and replacement foods, you can start trying to work them into your weekly routine. Don't try to make a dozen new recipes a week, unless you're really into cooking. That can wear you out and become a little disheartening, especially if you try to get too fancy. Settle for one new recipe a week, at first, and keep the rest of your meals safe and simple. Try to prepare a few things ahead of time and freeze them. We've had a lot of luck doing Chris' pancakes that way. Then we just microwave them as needed. You can do that with cupcakes and cookies, too.

The main idea is to surround your family with lots of good, healthy foods that everyone can eat, and to keep as few as possible of the foods your food-sensitive child can't eat in the house. That doesn't mean no one can eat cookies or ice cream if you have a celiac kid or a casein kid in the house. But that also doesn't mean safe snacks can't be just as tasty. And with all we've learned about "traditional" American food, the allergen-free stuff is probably better for you, anyway.

Ready, Set, Rotate!

Consider using a "rotation" diet for the whole family. Rotation diets are a good way to keep your diet varied and healthy by arranging meals in such a way that no one food or item from the same food family is eaten more than (ideally) once every four to seven days.

For instance, if you choose a four-day rotation diet and you eat something from the legume family on Monday—say lima beans—you can't have any legumes again until Thursday or Friday. Instead, you might eat from the cabbage family on Tuesday and then from the nightshade

> *My favorite gluten-free lunches or snacks are sandwiches made out of made out of wheat free pancakes and 'personal pan pizza's' with rice soft tacos as the crust."*—Nicole, 12

family (that's potatoes or tomatoes) on Wednesday and that will bring you to Thursday when you can have some succotash with limas again.

You can be as strict or lax with this idea as you like. You can have the same dishes, if you like, and just vary the ingredients from time to time; for instance, use rice flour in a recipe one day, and then try garfava (garbanzo and fava beans) flour in a similar recipe another day. A rotation diet is just an orderly way of diversifying your diet.

And if you or someone in your family is on a limited diet anyway, it's a good way of reducing the chances of it becoming even more limited by eating too much of any one food and causing a new intolerance. Sometimes, foods that cause mild problems may cease to cause problems at all when rotated. It's thought that putting more time between the ingestion of some foods gives our immune system a rest, and that might well be the case.

Ideally, you should be able to combine a rotation diet with your seven to fourteen day menu plans without too much trouble. If that still sounds like too much work, then just keep the idea of rotating foods every two to four days in the back of your mind as a healthy concept while you plan your meals. Remember the mantra: *Diversity is Good!*

Plan What You Eat, and Eat What You Plan
Now you're pretty much set to give it a shot. With a list of all

the foods you can use and a list of recipes you like by your side, make a seven-day plan for breakfast, lunch, and dinner.

As you can see from my own, (quite honestly) reproduced menu plan on the next page, I don't rotate nearly as often as I could. We tend to use rice quite a bit during the week, in a variety of forms. Then again, sometimes we'll go several days without it. I try to stay conscious of the fact that it's easy for us to use rice too often. While we also use beans a lot, they're not all in the same family, so we don't worry too much about that. I also tend to use leftovers from dinner within two or three days for lunch-time fare. Overall, I think our meals are varied and interesting. But it does take a little bit of work to get us beyond two weeks with reasonable variety.

Remember, too, that your meal plans will be influenced by your family's likes and dislikes, as well as cultural and regional influences. For example, since we live in Florida and I'm of Hispanic descent, our meals have a Cuban influence. Families living in the Southwest might favor dishes made with green chiles while those living in the South might favor grits. The point is, a good, varied diet is possible regardless of where you live, so develop your meal plans according to what you like.

Notice that during this week we had pancakes twice. However, on Thursday they were made from rice flour; on Friday they were made from potatoes. Same dish, different ingredients.

Chris' snacks and desserts typically consist of fruit, wheat-free cookies sometimes, yogurt or frozen yogurt, or trail mixes. One treat he really likes is Asian rice crackers with hummus—how's *that* for ethnic variety? Chris gets his own little hummus dish and we use a bigger dish of hummus to dip our flatbread in. If we mix and match wheat-free and "regular" foods, we always make sure Chris has his own servings in separate dishes to avoid cross contamination.

My Family's Weekly Menu

	Breakfast	Lunch	Dinner
Sunday	WF corn flakes Orange juice	Rice/Black beans Water	WF meatloaf Mashed potatoes Green beans Water
Monday	Rice pancakes Maple syrup Soy milk	Lean turkey, Succotash Water	Soft (corn) tacos Refried beans Corn chips Water
Tuesday	WF toast Rice cereal Soy milk	Fruit salad Yogurt Water	Cube steak Rice Black beans Fried plantains Water
Wednesday	Eggs Hash browns Orange juice	Tacos Refried beans Water	Grilled chicken Baked potatoes Peas Water
Thursday	Rice pancakes Soy milk	Cube steak Rice Fried plantains, Water	Cuban picadillo* Black beans Water
Friday	Potato pancakes Orange juice	Grilled chicken Baked beans Water	WF pasta Salad WF garlic bread Water
Saturday	WF cornflakes Soy milk	Rice/black beans Water	Baked chicken Sweet potato chips Lima beans Water

WF=wheat-free   *See recipe for Picadillo in Chapter 11.

You'll notice that water is our beverage for much of the day. It's what we drink between meals, too. I think water is the finest beverage ever invented. Children don't fill up on it when they eat, it keeps them hydrated between meals, and they don't get empty calories from juice or sodas. It's interesting to see our reactions to soda and other sweet beverages now that they're older and have grown up drinking mostly water. They don't like the taste of sodas at all, and they typically reject the sweet drinks guzzled by other kids in favor of water. And, they naturally limit their intake of sweets, cakes, and cookies. I think that's evidence that kids can become "hooked" on good foods as easily as they can on bad ones.

Cross Contamination
This is probably a good place to bring up the issue of cross-contamination and maintaining a safe cooking environment. Many food sensitivities can be triggered by even minimal exposure to the target food.

The best way to avoid problems is to be vigilant about hand washing, counter cleaning, and using separate utensils and storage containers. Always use the same containers for your food sensitive child's safe foods. Fix any special items for their meals first, then prepare everything else. Then, clean countertops, ovens, and grills thoroughly so they're ready next time. Always wash your hands a lot in the kitchen—and insist others do as well. Besides being a plain old good habit—especially with rising threats of salmonella and other food-borne bacteria issues—it helps avoid cross-contamination.

Allergy-Free Goes High Tech
And here's a high-tech assist. Got a computer? Go online and find a veritable living library of health and nutrition information plus a huge selection of software for menu analysis and recipe planning. Here is a brief description of these products.[94]

---

[94] For a full report on these products, contact Savory Palate, Inc. 8174 S. Holly, #404, Littleton, CO 80122-4004, and ask for Home Menu/Recipe Planning Software Report.

Product[95]	Description
On-Line Analyzers	
www.MealsforYou.com	Free. Search recipes by ingredients, nutrients, category, special diets (diabetes, vegetarians—not allergies)
www.KitchenLink.com	Free. 10,000 Internet cooking links. Nutrient data, substitutions, recipes. Some allergy information.
http://skyisland.com/OnlineResources/ cookbook/cookbook.html	Free. Partly developed by FAST. Allergy-specific recipes and substitutions at this online cookbook.
Celiac UPC Database http://www.brandtbeach.com/celiac/upc/in dex.html (Work in progress, not complete)	Free. For use by celiacs to determine if a product is gluten-free, based on UPC product code. Access online or by telephone or hand-held PC.
Home Recipe/Menu Planning	
NutriGenie software http://pages.prodigy.com/CA/nutrigenie/ home.html	$30-$50. Meal planners for rotation diets, diabetes, immune deficiency.
Zing Solutions FAP AID Also see web site at http://zingsolutions.com/food	Regularly $200, *$160 if you mention this book*. Background information and reported reactions to allergens, foods; food families, cross-reactions; additives, preservatives, and more.
MasterCook by SierraOriginals http://www.sierra.com/	$10-$40, depending on version. Thousands of recipes, categorized by meal, ingredients, nutrition, etc. Can customize for special diet. Menu planning capability.
Nutritionist Five by First DataBank http://www.firstdatabank.com/nutrition/nu trifive.html	$500. Used by dietitians and corporations.
The Food Processor by ESHA http://www.esharesearch.com/	$700. Used by dietitians and corporations.

---

[95] This list is not intended to be complete, but to represent a good cross-section of software.

149

Volume Cooking

One of the best techniques I've found for meeting all our needs in one fell swoop is "volume" cooking. I try to make enough during one cooking session to use as leftovers within a couple of days, as ingredients in other meals, or that I can freeze and use later. I especially like freezing foods. When Chris was little, I would make up his homemade baby food and freeze it in ice cube trays, which made perfect baby-sized serving portions.

When I make Chris' rice flour pancakes, I make them on the griddle first and freeze them by the dozen. Every other morning or so, I can microwave however many he wants for breakfast. I can also make up loaves of gluten-free breads and freeze those to use as needed. Wheat-free meatballs freeze well, too, and can be used with wheat-free pasta meals or on their own with vegetable side dishes.

Tracey makes up mixes in advance, as well. "Mix up dry ingredients for breads, etc. and store them in the freezer until you need to bake. Then just add wet ingredients. Mix flour mixes ...one day a month or at whatever interval is needed."

Sometimes I can plan meals around leftovers. If I make cornbread one night, I can make a nice gluten-free meatloaf with some of that same cornbread the following night. And then I can use the meatloaf in sandwiches or for lunch the day after that. I can also crumble leftover cornbread and freeze it to use later for recipes that require breadcrumbs. If I make picadillo (a Spanish style, seasoned beef dish), which Chris loves, I can use picadillo leftovers for tacos a night or two later. I like to think of myself as culinary efficiency expert. It's like playing Connect Four™ in the kitchen, making everything fit neatly together.

Just remember to label everything properly when you store your finished products. Once, I volume-cooked Chris' pancakes and regular pancakes and forgot to label the freezer bags. The next morning, I stood at the freezer door staring at the two bags long enough to get cold before I finally threw both of them out and started over. Chris' pancakes taste quite like the "real" thing and after nibbling samples from one bag and then the other, I just couldn't tell the difference. So I erred on the side of safety and never forgot to label anything properly again.

Kitchen Zen

Part of what I've learned from all this "special" cooking is that it's not all that special. It's a return, however forced, to a regular, ordinary part of life that many of us have lost touch with for a variety of reasons. Often—and I know quite frequently out of necessity—outside work limits our time in the kitchen and meaningful mealtime get-togethers. We speed through breakfast, rush kids to daycare or school, hurry to work, wolf down lunch, careen home for end-of-day activities and chores, rush through dinner, throw everyone in baths and into bed, and then start all over again the next day.

We've actually reached a point in our society where celebrities make as many public service TV commercials imploring families to take time to eat together as they do imploring us not to take drugs. Even higher medicine has turned its resources to studying American eating habits. In "Family Dinner and Diet Quality Among Older Children and Adolescents", a study recently published in the Journal of the American Medical Association (JAMA)[96], researchers contend that families that eat together stay healthy together.

Wrote the researchers," Our results show that family dinner is associated with some healthful dietary patterns. Increasing frequency of family dinner was associated with higher consumption of fruits and vegetables and several beneficial nutrients, including fiber, folate, calcium, iron, and vitamins B6, B12, C, and E."

---

[96] Family dinner and diet quality among older children and dolescents, Journal of the American Medical Association, Vol. 9 No. 3, March 2000

151

The researchers went on to conclude that families that dined together regularly also seemed to have a higher concept of health than other families. Health and diet were frequently topics of conversation at the dinner table, and these children often seemed well versed in health issues.

The point is that, in what may be something of a mixed blessing, food sensitivities throw a wrench in the staccato clockwork of our days and force us to take stock of a fundamental life issue—the way we meet one of our most basic daily needs, nourishment. American eating, like much of American life itself, is rooted in the convenient.

Eating in America, which was once a major social endeavor—and in many parts of the world remains so—has been reduced to "power meals" and "fast food." Our reverence of and appreciation for the fruits of the earth, our connection with the very essence of life itself, with nourishment, has been severed in our headlong rush to get to wherever it is we're in a hurry to go.

Whether this same frenetic rush has anything to do with the increasing prevalence of food sensitivities in the U.S.; whether it drives our hurry to feed our children solid foods in infancy to get them along the road to maturity faster, or fuels our predisposition to eat a lot of the same, mass produced, allergen laden prepared foods and thus create our own food sensitivities, is probably better left to private speculation. What's done is done.

Take Time and Smell the Garlic

What we can do here is take the cards we've been dealt and use the opportunity to assess the hand we now hold. Attitude is the key to the game from here on out, and the attitude we adopt in dealing with food sensitivity can set the tone for a lifetime of health and well-being. One way you can look at the task set before you is that you now have an unparalleled excuse to slow down. The label reading alone is going to take hours!

But it's the time in the kitchen that offers the most rewards, nutritionally and spiritually. I know it can seem like a stretch here, but bear with me. Time anywhere can be redeeming, but time spent with food—holding it, washing it, peeling and slicing it, seasoning, marinating, smelling and feeling and tasting it—can literally re-anchor your life.

Our ancestral roots are nomadic, following herds and gathering foods found along the way. It was agriculture that led to civilization, to the development of society. The ability to cultivate our own food gave us the ability to live richer, broader lives. Food marks our celebrations and the rituals of our lives, and yet we never really think about it—unless we can get it out of a box or a bag and it's sweet and rich and sticky.

Now you have a food-sensitive child. Now you have to look at the food you eat. Now you have to reduce it down to the bare essentials, to its purest forms, distilled to a non-allergenic essence of simplicity. Behold food! From the ground, from trees, from vines and marshy fields and golden meadows. It is beautiful! The textured skin of a carrot, the earthy odor of a baking potato, the fragrance of a smooth-skinned apple, the savory aroma of seasoned rice simmering quietly on the stove.

As you learn to prepare foods your food-sensitive child and your whole family can enjoy, take the opportunity to engage in a little kitchen Zen. There is elegance to pure, wholesome foods that nothing in a box or a bag can ever approach. You don't have to be the Galloping Gourmet to appreciate that elegance. Use your kitchen time, whether it's daily, or just one day a week you set aside, to regain time for yourself and for your family, and a sense of beauty and richness that will nourish you far outside the walls of your kitchen.

Summing it All Up

- *Make family meals everyone can enjoy* **instead of "special"**

153

meals for your food-sensitive child and "regular" meals for the rest of the family. Make food a non-issue at your house.

- *When beginning menu planning, first explore your options.* Be creative; think "outside the box" as you search out new foods to try. And try everything with (hopefully contagious) enthusiasm.

- *Use Menu Planning to assist in developing some sort of rotation diet.* The more you can vary your meals, and the longer time you can put in between the consumption of particular foods and food families, the more safely you can alleviate, and sometimes eliminate, food sensitivities.

- *Plan what you eat and eat what you plan!* Try organizing your meals into one and two week Menu Planning charts for ease of preparation and to help you use leftovers and other foods more efficiently.

- *Volume Cooking* is a good way to minimize your overall time in the kitchen preparing special foods. Cook and freeze things like pancakes, meatballs, and other foods and then use as needed.

- *The family that eats together stays healthy together.* Cooking at home and eating regular meals together can improve everyone's health and quality of life.

- *Practice Kitchen Zen:* Get back in touch with food as the source of nourishment for spirit, mind and body by connecting with it in a new and mindful way.

Chapter IX
Grocery Shopping: A Label Primer

Even if we agree that becoming one with your kitchen is the next best thing to entering Nirvana, there's just no way around the fact that unless you've got your own big kitchen garden you have to go grocery shopping with some frequency. And that may require the patience of Job more than the Zen of Buddha.

"On my first trip to the grocery store," recalled Danna, "I set out with a great attitude. After all, I'm a well-educated, intelligent young woman—what could be so difficult about reading a few labels? Three hours later, tears smearing mascara all over my face, I left with three bags of Fritos™. I was sure I would never be able to feed him again."

Of course, Danna found out she could indeed feed Tyler. The key here is one you're no doubt familiar with by now—education. There's no substitute for knowledge when it comes to reading labels, and you're going to be reading lots of labels unless you're just buying produce. And reading labels can be like speaking in tongues!

Allergens can come cloaked in a variety of tongue-twisting nomenclatures, and even if you know them all you can still be confounded in your efforts to find safe food by the fact that not all ingredients are always listed anyway. That's one reason that the fewer ingredients a product has—and the more pronounceable and recognizable—the less chance you have of endangering your food-sensitive child's health.

An FDA ABC
The Food and Drug Administration (FDA) has come a long way in what it requires of food manufacturers in terms of labeling. And, to its credit, the food industry has come a long way in compliance and in its appreciation of and respect for customer

155

demands for better and more precise content information. But while laws about nutritional labeling and claims are quite precise and far-reaching—right down to the location of the label on the package and the size of the type used—regulations regarding ingredient lists are more vague.

Additives in our foods are many, varied, and frequently hidden.[97] The FDA says they're used, among other things, to "keep foods wholesome," an intriguing thought since one would think "wholesome" things don't need anything added, just by virtue of their being wholesome. Mostly, though, additives are used to preserve foods, enhance appearance and consistency, and improve texture and taste.

Typical additives are grouped under such headings as:
- φ *Emulsifiers* to give foods consistent texture and help hold them together,
- φ *Stabilizers and thickeners* for uniform texture,
- φ *Anti-caking agents* to help things like salt flow freely,
- φ *Vitamins and minerals* to improve nutritional content (and sometimes often to hide the fact that the item wouldn't be considered nutritional otherwise!) These can often sound scarier than they are: alphatocopherol, for example, is just another name for Vitamin E.
- φ *Preservatives* to help retard spoilage caused by mold, bacteria, fungi, yeast and air,
- φ *Leavening agents* to control acidity or alkalinity in baked goods,
- φ *Natural and artificial flavors*, used for flavor enhancement, are often clumped together on labels, and
- φ *Spices* for obvious reasons.

As of 1993[98], the FDA began requiring that ingredients for "all standardized foods" be listed on labels, including labels on meat

---

[97] Ruth Winter's "Consumer's Dictionary for Additives," (see Bibliography for complete information) is an excellent resource which lists all additives with background information. The FAP AID (Food Additive and Preservative Allergy and Intolerance Database), by Zing Solutions, also is an excellent resource, with additional information on cross reactivity.
[98] Food and Drug Administration data from FDA website and nutritional labeling handbook. See reference section for addresses and additional information.

and poultry products. Ingredients are listed in order of predominance by weight; i.e., the ingredient weighing the most in a product is listed first, the one weighing least is listed last. FDA-certified color additives, were also required to be listed by name, rather than collectively under the headings "flavorings," "spices, or "colorings." Required that is, *except,* in butter, cheese, and ice cream. And that was for all colorings *except* for caramel, paprika, and beet juice, which can be listed as "artificial colors" without being specifically identified.

And that is the principal problem with FDA guidelines regarding ingredient listings: there are a *lot* of exceptions. As of the 1990 ruling, caseinates have to be identified as a milk derivative, but not whey, or lactobumin or any of the other milk derivatives we discussed earlier. And non-dairy creamers are *still* labeled non-dairy, despite the occurrence of dairy by-products such as caseinates.

Another problem area is protein hydrolysates, or hydrolyzed vegetable proteins. Hydrolyzed proteins are proteins that are broken down by an acid or enzyme into amino acids and which are added to foods as leavening agents, stabilizers, thickeners, flavorings, flavor enhancers and nutrients, to name just a few of their uses. Typically, vegetable proteins used this way have simply been identified as "flavorings" or "natural flavors."

In 1993, the FDA declared that protein hydrolysates added to foods as flavorings function as "flavor enhancers" and must therefore be declared by their common, or usual, name, and that the source of the protein thus used must also be identified. That meant that the vague "hydrolyzed vegetable protein" had to be identified as "hydrolyzed corn protein," or "hydrolyzed casein," as the case may be.
From a food sensitivity perspective, this sounds like label heaven. Clearly, the uniform labeling of products containing sulfites has been of enormous benefit to those sensitive to sulfiting agents. Unfortunately, I still see a lot of "hydrolyzed

157

vegetable protein" on labels I read. Occasionally, I'll come across a parenthetical (corn) or (potato) reference, but not very often. That same ruling called for "voluntary inclusion" of the actual source of various sweeteners. Instead of "dextrose," food manufacturers could label the ingredient more precisely as "corn sugar monohydrate." But in all honesty, how often have you seen that listing? And "modified food starch" has yet to be clearly identified on packaging.

Effective this year (2000), however, proper identification of protein hydrolysates becomes mandatory and perhaps we'll be able to better understand what's in our foods. According to the 2000 ruling, food manufacturers will have to declare the source of these proteins (corn, wheat, potato, etc.). The new law states specifically, "the source of all protein hydrolysates—regardless of use—will now have to be identified." And "caseinate will have to be identified as a milk derivative when used in foods claiming to be non-dairy".[99] Such requirements leave little to the manufacturers' imaginations regarding how such items are identified on labels, and a lot less to our imaginations as well!

Standardized Foods
As a rule, the FDA requires ingredient lists on all "standardized foods." The FDA acknowledges the following product categories of standardized foods:

Milk and cream • Cheeses and related products • Frozen desserts • Bakery products • Cereal flours and related products • Macaroni and noodle products • Canned fruits • Canned fruit juices • Fruit butters • Jellies, and jams or preserves • Fruit pies • Canned vegetables • Vegetable juices • Frozen vegetables • Eggs and egg products • Fish and shellfish • Cacao products (for example, cocoa, chocolate) • Tree nut and peanut products • Margarine • Sweeteners and table syrups • Food dressings and flavorings (for example, mayonnaise, salad dressing, vanilla flavoring)

That is, of course, all standardized foods *except* those served in hospital cafeterias, airplanes, food service vendors—including

---

[99] Celiac Support Page, March 2000

mall cookie counters, sidewalk vendors and vending machines, ready-to-eat foods prepared on-site at bakeries, delis, and candy stores—foods shipped in bulk (as long as it's not sold in that form to consumers), medical foods, plain coffee and tea, some spices, and "other foods that contain *no significant amounts of any nutrients.*"[100] Foods produced by businesses employing fewer than 100 full time employees can claim exemptions from labeling requirements as well.

Also, the FDA exempts "trace ingredients" from being listed if an ingredient is an "incidental additive and has no function or technical effect in the finished product." (Regardless of what kind of function or technical effect it might have on the consumer!) Sulfites, for instance, are considered "incidental" if present at less than 10 parts per meter.

Alternative fats and oils (that insidious "and/or" listing) are allowed only when foods contain relatively small amounts of added fat or oil in foods where these are not the primary ingredient and only if the manufacturer is unable to predict which fat or oil ingredient will be used (which can be troublesome if you're sensitive to the one the manufacturer ends up using!)

Spices, artificial flavors, and natural flavors can be declared using either specific common or usual names or simply by the designations "spices," "flavor," "natural flavor" or "artificial flavor," without further disclosure. Vegetable powders are supposed to be identified by their "specific" name, such as "celery powder."

So now that you know all this, what can you do with it? Well, you can definitely stick to the produce department as much as possible, but you can also shop more wisely when you understand just what—and what doesn't—go into FDA food labeling.

---

[100] The italics are mine, with the thought in mind that while the nutrient content may not be "significant" by FDA standards, the ingredient content may nonetheless be significant enough to cause problems for some people.

Hitting the Aisles

Obviously, you'll probably find the safest items in your local produce market and health food store. Of course, it's just as important to read health food store labels as grocery store labels, but you'll probably find the reading lighter and more comforting!

You'll probably find that there are some items you can only get in a health food store and some that you can get in grocery stores. We simply stock up on special things during our once-a-month trip to the health food store.

Talk to the Management

And strike up a rapport with store managers. They can be your best allies when it comes to the foods you need or want to buy. If you like a particular line of food, be sure to tell the manager. If there's one you wish your store carried, tell the manager and explain why. If you've got friends who feel the same way, make sure they talk to the manager, too. If a store suddenly stops carrying a food you find helpful or enjoy, make sure you express your disappointment.

Store and department managers are an often overlooked resource who really want to hear from customers, and typically are quite responsive to consumer needs and inquiries. If we don't keep stores informed about our needs, they won't be able to meet them. And if they know that food sensitivities are an issue, they'll be more conscious of that issue when making their buying decisions for their store.

Label Changes

One of the things that can change without notice is that label you've just learned to read. New preservatives are always being developed or recipes changed, and sometimes the overall packaging won't reflect these changes immediately or clearly. So, get in the habit of reading the label every time, even if it's something you purchase regularly. And familiarize yourself with the most basic additives and ingredients in the foods you use, so that you can recognize changes quickly.

Subsequent chapters cover food families, ingredient synonyms, and substitutions. But for now, let's just look at some basic "safe shopping" issues and how to apply your new label savvy in both the health food store and the grocery store.

Always Read the Label

Now that you're an expert and can go down those food aisles like a general inspecting his troops, you might be pleasantly surprised. A few companies are now including "Allergy Alerts" on their packaging.[101] Some products, like Chex Mix™, for instance, will include, in bold type beneath the ingredients, a list of any potentially allergy-causing ingredients in the product. Chex Mix™, by the way, has almost all of them: soy, milk, wheat, corn, and peanuts. But at least they warn you.

Quite recently, Baskin Robbins™ Ice Cream employed new ingredient labels on their ice cream display windows in some areas. Now, along with the flavor name and description, the company is including information about potential allergens in each flavor, and even gluten is noted!

Allergy alerts, though, are purely voluntary. They're not required by law, and they're typically used only if the possible allergen is not already listed as an official ingredient; i.e. they're

---

[101] The Food Allergy Network (FAN) provides consumer "allergy alerts," notifying members of recalls and ingredient changes that may not be obvious at the store.

161

named only if there is the possibility of inadvertent contamination through manufacturing or packing procedures.[102]

You'll also find some disappointments. Allergy alerts aside, you still have the vagaries of "vegetable proteins" or "vegetable oil" or "food starch", as well as possibly allergenic foods masked as flavorings, seasonings, or spices. And, if you're looking at foods marketed internationally, then you're looking at even less regulation than in the U.S. Much of what's disclosed on U.S. food packages isn't required on imported items.

There are two things you can do to hedge your bets when it comes to any of these uncertainties. First, you can put the suspect product back on the shelf and get something else. And second, you can contact the manufacturer of the product and ask specific questions about the ingredients. Almost all major U.S. food manufacturers have information numbers printed on their packages, and almost all of them are cooperative in answering food related questions. You can also ask the larger companies, like Kraft™ or Heinz™ or Nabisco™, for lists of their gluten-free or casein-free products, or for lists of peanut containing products, or any other type of allergen you're screening for, and they'll send it out to you.

FAST (Food Allergy Survivors Together) suggests these tips for contacting manufacturers.

1) *Be wary of quick answers*. Representatives who give over-confident, quick answers are likely not aware of the fact that the flavorings can be a food product. They may just be looking at the same label you are, instead of trying to find out what the flavorings and accidental ingredients are.

2) *Always assume that the person on the other end of the phone knows less about labeling than you do.*

---

[102] Allergy Network of Calgary, affiliated with Allergy Asthma Information Association, 16531 – 114 Street, Edmonton, AB T5X 3V6. http://cgi.cadvision.com/~allergy/index.html

162

3) *Ask for it in writing.* FAST members have mentioned that asking for this information in writing rather than over the phone results in more careful replies. Frequently, companies will include a disclaimer in the e-mail or in a letter such as "but we cannot guarantee that it will be free of..." So they leave it to your discretion to decide whether or not to risk trying the product. But that's still better than glibly being led to believe something is safe when it's not.

4) *When calling manufacturers, ask what is IN the product rather than what is NOT in the product.* If you phrase your inquiry as, "My son is allergic to milk. Is there any milk in this product?" the phone representative may look at the natural flavorings or accidental additives and not realize that words such as casein, lactalbumin, and whey mean milk. You may get inaccurate information.

5) *Remember that the flavoring contents can change any day without a difference in the label!* Follow up the call regularly if you decide to use the product. We can't be reminded too often that the ingredients in manufactured foods can change at any time. Always read the labels of products you buy regularly, so you don't get lulled into a sense of false security

Besides providing you with the most up-to-date information on products, your inquiries will help keep food sensitivities as a "top-of-the-mind" issue for food manufacturers.

Red Flags
In addition to being a label expert, you've also got to know your way around a store. You don't want to founder in red flag areas like bulk bins and bakeries. Bulk bins can be tempting, especially in health food stores or the health food sections of grocery stores. They *look* healthy and appealing, and you can choose just what you need. But a word of caution is in order. First, there's no way to tell how pure the bulk product is. FDA labeling is certainly not required under these circumstances. Second,

the danger of cross-contamination is high. Scoops get moved between bins in such situations, and bins can be used for different items and may not be cleaned between uses.

Bakeries should raise additional flags, and not just for the gluten intolerant who shouldn't be there in the first place. If you're sensitive to peanuts or other nuts, you should avoid bakery items that have been on display near other items that may have nuts in them. Cross contamination is of major concern in the bakery environment, and widely handled or loosely packaged foods should be avoided. As a rule, you should stick to baked prepackaged foods that are clearly labeled and tightly packaged.

The deli area should raise some flags, too. The danger of cross contamination with various ingredients in various foods is high at the deli. Meat slicers, for instance, are used for slicing both cheese and meat. And it's probably not a good idea to purchase some take out deli foods that may have been prepared on counters which may have been contaminated by other allergens.

Hidden Allergens

The biggest red flag raiser is one of which we're rarely aware: hidden allergens. Hidden allergens are just that—hidden— usually in a food we would consider safe to ingest. Hidden allergens typically result from cross contamination of foods from serving utensils, storage facilities, food preparation areas, and food manufacturing equipment.

Another hidden allergen that can lurk unseen and unbidden in labels occurs when manufacturers use previously manufactured products in the creation of a secondary product.[103] For instance, mayonnaise used in making a new product may not result in the listing of mayonnaise or egg for that product, especially if the mayonnaise accounts for less than two percent of the ingredients. Some margarines labeled "100% corn oil" may also con-

---

[103] Steinman, HA. Hidden allergens in foods. Journal of Allergy and Clinical Immunology 1996; 98 (2):241-250

tain skim milk powder. Similarly, seemingly non-dairy drinks for those unable to tolerate milk can be milk with lactase enzyme in it.

Sometimes egg can be a hidden allergen cloaked as "binder" or "protein" or "emulsifier." Soy will not be listed specifically as such if it is used for "texturizing" food. When pineapple, milk casein, or hydrolyzed soy protein are used for flavoring, the label may say "natural flavors" or "flavoring."

The Food Allergy Survivors Together (FAST) support group says that unlisted ingredients in foods can cause problems, despite manufacturers claims to the contrary. FAST also points out that with 5 million Americans having food allergies, (that's more people than have epilepsy, hemophilia, emphysema, and multiple sclerosis combined!), it could only behoove manufacturers to be more specific on their labels. Especially since we all know by now—when in doubt, leave it on the shelf. If we knew what those "flavorings" were and they were safe, we'd certainly be more likely to buy it. Until manufacturers figure that out, though, we have to continue to be careful—and diligent. Remember the food sensitivity battle cry: *Never Assume Anything*!

"We shouldn't try to predict what natural flavorings will be in products," notes Melissa Taylor, head of FAST, "because often we are wrong. I would have never guessed that a [piece of] bacon I was eating had 'natural flavorings' consisting of *grains*—I assumed it meant spices!"

Reactions to Hidden Ingredients
According to FAST, there are a few ways you might be able to tell if you're having a reaction to unlabeled food ingredients. If you've eaten a new food and all the ingredients seemed okay, but you have telltale reactions within 72 hours after eating the food, there may be a hidden item that you're reacting to. If it's a food you've eaten before and you're having a problem, double-check the label. Maybe you missed something. Sometimes it's

165

an issue of cross contamination. If there are vaguely named ingredients on the label, call the manufacturer for clarification.

To find out about hidden ingredients in products, says FAST, specifically ask the manufacturer what a product's natural flavorings are made of. It may take them a while to figure this out, and some manufacturers will not take the time to help you. Still others will take the time, even if it means returning your phone call at their cost. Find a manufacturer you can trust for reliable information. Remember—the answers that take a long time to receive are often a lot more reliable than fast answers!

"Some manufacturers will only answer questions on hidden ingredients if you agree to their rules (which is nevertheless better than the manufacturers who refuse on all counts!)," says Taylor. She says some manufacturers will request a complete listing of your allergens, so they can compare that to the ingredients in a product and let you know whether there may be a hidden item to which you're reacting.

"If you decide to go this route, it requires through-the-mail correspondence. Make a complete listing of all of your allergens and their alternative names. This can take a long time if you have multiple food allergies! But once you get it finished you can keep a copy, saved on your computer hard-drive, or photocopy it. Include a self addressed stamped envelope if you can— it might better guarantee a reply. "If you use email for this type of correspondence, says FAST, remember to send yourself a copy of your email so you can keep records."

"If you do get sick from unlabeled ingredients," suggests Taylor, "It may be a good idea to write to the manufacturer and let them know about it (after you have determined it was definitely an unlabeled ingredient—call and ask first). Your diligence in doing so may keep another person from getting sick." Here's a good sample letter to a manufacturer:

"Dear Sir or Madam:

My child is sensitive to corn. We enjoy your products, but need to select foods carefully for our food sensitive child.

May we please have a list of your corn free products? Or, if that is unavailable, could you please advise us as to the exact content of the following foods? (List here exactly which items you need to have ingredients for.)

I've attached an information sheet with this letter to give you a brief overview of this type of sensitivity.

Thanks so much for your time and attention, and we look forward to continuing to enjoy your products.

Getting There from Here

Now, there's just not much you can do about some of these issues, other than simply be aware that they exist. You already know that the fewer ingredients a product has, the safer it probably is. And you also know what terms to be suspicious of, depending on what sensitivities your child has. Now, I could make an extensive list here of what you *can't* buy for your food-sensitive child, but I think it will be a lot more helpful and certainly less distressing, to know what you can buy *instead*.

If Someone is Wheat Sensitive[104]

⊘ AVOID	☑ USE instead
Calcium caseinate or Sodium caseinate (contains MSG, which is safe if made in U.S.).	*Calcium phosphate, calcium chloride.*
Dextrins.[105]	*Maltodextrin is okay.[106]*

---

[104] From the Safe and Forbidden lists of the Celiac Support Page. Used by permission of Scott Adams. See resource section for address.

[105] Dextrins are incompletely hydrolyzed starch. They are prepared by dry heating corn, waxy maize, waxy milo, potato, arrowroot, WHEAT, rice, tapioca, or sago starches, or by dry heating the starches after: (1) Treatment with safe and suitable alkalis, acids, or pH control agents and (2) drying the acid or alkali treated starch. Therefore, unless you know the source, you must avoid dextrin.

[106] Maltodextrin is prepared as a white powder or concentrated solution by partial hydrolysis of cornstarch or potato starch with safe and suitable acids and enzymes. (1) Maltodextrin, when

If Someone is Wheat Sensitive (continued)

⊘ AVOID	☑ USE instead
Hydrolyzed vegetable protein.	*Products where protein source is identified as non-wheat.*
Hydrolyzed plant protein.	*Plant proteins where plant is specifically identified.*
Malt.	*Maltodextrin is okay. See footnote 106.*
Modified food starch.	*Starch source must be specifically identified.*
Mono and di-glycerides. [107]	*Check with manufacturer.*
Rice malt (can contain barley or Koji).	*Rice or other flours, without malt.*
And these grain products:	***Vary the use of these:***
Barley, (wheat) bran, couscous, drum wheat triticum, einkorn, graham flour, kamut, rye, semolina, spelt, wheat germ, wheat triticum durum. (See footnotes 7 and 30 for a discussion of oats.)	*Amaranth, arrowroot, bean flours, corn flour, corn meal, cornstarch, millet, nut flours, potato flour, potato starch, quinoa, rice flour, sorghum flour, soy flour, tapioca flour.*

A Note on Vinegar: You may wonder why vinegar does not appear in these charts. Except for the malt varieties, vinegar is considered safe for celiacs. The single word "vinegar" on a label indicates apple cider vinegar. Typically, distilled white vinegar is made from corn. Wheat is rarely used in the distillation process and even if it were, the gluten peptides cannot survive the distillation process. It's possible that vinegar may cause reactions in some people. If so, it's likely due to a sensitivity to vinegar itself and is solved by avoiding it. The same goes for vanilla extract or flavoring, both often avoided by the gluten-sensitive, but considered safe by researchers who say the

---

listed on food sold in the U.S., must be (per FDA regulation) made from corn or potato. This rule does NOT apply to vitamin or mineral supplements/medications. (2) Donald Kasarda Ph.D., a USDA research chemist specializing in grain proteins, found that all maltodextrins in the U.S. are made from cornstarch, using enzymes that are NOT derived from wheat, rye, barley, or oats. On that basis he believes that celiacs need not avoid maltodextrins, though he cautions that there is no guarantee that a manufacturer won't change processes to use wheat starch or gluten-based enzymes in the future. (3) May 1997 Sprue-Nik News, Celiac Support Page.

[107] These can contain wheat in the U.S. Typically derived of fats, carbohydrate chains may be used as a binding substance in their preparation, which are usually corn or wheat.

gluten peptides can't survive the distillation process. Imitation vanilla is a synthetic product made from vanillin, the main flavoring component of vanilla, and may be made from wood pulp by-products, again not an issue for the wheat-sensitive.[108] Always remember, though: When in doubt, contact the manufacturer.

If Someone is Sensitive to Milk[109]

⊘ AVOID	☑ USE instead
Milk solids ("curds"), whey.	Almond, oat, rice, and soy milk.
Casein (sodium caseinate, most commonly).	Avoid all caseinates.
Lactose (sodium lactylate, frequently lactalbumin and other names that begin with lact.	Galactose (lactose by-product) Most milk-allergic people have no trouble with galactose.
"Natural" ingredients.	Ask manufacturer, or use only when clearly identified as safe.
Hydrolyzed vegetable protein.[110]	Check with manufacturer for exact source of protein.
"Non-dairy" anything, including Cool Whip.[111]	Read label to determine true extent of "non-dairy."
Kosher pareve desserts.[112]	Most, but not all, pareve foods are ok. See below.
Canned tuna.[113]	Low sodium in spring water (e.g., Starkist and Trader Joe).
Some chocolate candy.[114]	Kosher pareve chocolates

[108] "Is Vinegar Safe for Celiacs?," Gluten-Free Living, September/October 1999, and "Are Natural and Artificial Flavorings Safe?", Gluten-Free Living, November/December 1999
[109] From the "No-Milk" page. See Resources for address
[110] For very sensitive, since processing phase may utilize casein.
[111] Non-dairy does not mean milk-free. It is a term used by the dairy industry to indicate less than 1/2 % milk by weight, which could mean fully as much casein as whole milk.
[112] Most pareve foods are okay, but occasionally milk-sensitive diners report trouble with desserts. Under most circumstances, Jewish dietary symbols on food packages are a reliable indicator of food content. If the product is dairy, it will frequently have a D or the word Dairy next to the kashrut (the K in the circle or a K in a star symbol). If it is pareve (made without milk, meat, or their derivatives) the word Pareve (or Parev) may appear near the symbol. Milchig, another dietary law term, also means made of or derived from milk or dairy products.
[113] Many brands contain "hydrolyzed caseinate".
[114] Dark or bittersweet chocolate may be run on same production line as milk chocolate, and risk of cross-contamination is high if YOUR chocolate bar comes from beginning of run.

If Someone is Sensitive to Milk (continued)

⊘ AVOID	☑ USE instead
Baked goods.[115]	*Unless certified safe through a known source, or homemade.*
Processed meats.[116]	*Check with manufacturer or buy non-processed meats only.*
Ice creams, dairy products.	*Vegan alternatives.*
Protein hydrolysates.	*Ask manufacturer for source.*

If Someone is Sensitive to Peanuts

⊘ AVOID	☑ USE instead
Mixed nuts.	*Nut sources you're sure of. Do not try to pick "safe" nuts from a container of mixed nuts.117*
Peanut Butter.	*Soy nut or almond butters.118*
Legumes.	*Check Food Families in Appendix.*

If Someone is Sensitive to Eggs

⊘ AVOID	☑ USE instead
Albumin, ovalbumin, globulin, livetin, ovomucin, ovomucoid, silici albuminate, vitellin, ovovitellin.	*Ask manufacturer if unsure.*
Powdered egg, dried egg yolk, egg white.	*Pureed flaxseeds, pureed fruit, tofu, commercial egg replacer.*
Egg noodles.	*Egg-free pastas like 100% corn, semolina, spelt, or quinoa.*
Milk puddings and custards.	*Egg-less custards and puddings.*
Pre- made pastries and breads.	*Make your own or special order or buy at health food store.*
Mayonnaise.	*Make your own egg-free version or use Nayonaise or Veganaise.*

---

[115] Nutrient value of flours, cereals, and baked goods is improved by Lysine-rich Sodium Caseinate.

[116] Sodium Caseinate helps bind processed meats (sausages, luncheon meats, liverwurst, meat loaf). It also acts as an emulsifier for fat.

[117] Unless you're one of the third of those sensitive to peanuts who also cannot eat tree nuts

[118] Be aware that nut butters may be run on the same lines as peanuts that are processed for peanut butter or other foods. Check with the manufacturer before using. See Footnote above.

If Someone is Sensitive to Corn

⊘ AVOID	☑ USE instead
Lecithins.	Ask manufacturer about source
Dextrose.[119]	Ask manufacturer about source.
Dextrin and maltodextrin.[120]	Potato starch or other thickener.
Caramel flavoring.[121]	Ask manufacturer or seek identified sources of flavoring.
Corn syrup.[122]	100% pure maple syrup, cane syrup, or beet sugars.
Fructose is usually made of high fructose corn syrup.	Sucrose or other known sweeteners like maple or beet
Invert syrup or sugar is enzymatically treated bulk corn sugars.	Cane sugar, maple syrups, agave nectar.
Cornstarch is added to most confectioners' sugars and baking powders to prevent clumping.	Use corn-free powdered sugar from Miss Roben's (See Vendors)
Food starch, modified food starch, vegetable gum/starch.[123]	Items where food starch source is specifically identified.
Malt, malt syrup or malt extract.[124]	Ask manufacturer for exact source.
Mono- and di-glycerides.[125]	Ask manufacturer for exact source.
Glucona delta lactone.[126]	Avoid.
Marshmallows can contain corn.	Ask manufacturer if corn-free.
Vanilla extract typically contains corn syrup.	Health food kind of vanilla extracts Some artificial vanilla (not "pure" vanilla extract) may be ok.
Xanthan gum.[127]	Guar gum, but may cause intestinal distress for celiacs.

[119] Dextrose can be a corn-based product and is used in cookies, ice cream and sports drinks. It is also used in French fries, fish sticks and potato puffs.

[120] Both of these are often made from cornstarch and are typically used in sauces, dressings, and ice cream as thickeners.

[121] Caramel flavoring can be made with corn syrup, as well as cane or beet sugar.

[122] Corn syrup is used in maple, nut and root beer flavorings for ice cream, ices, candies, baked good, soft drinks and fruit drinks.

[123] May be made of corn.

[124] Usually a red flag for the gluten intolerant, but as it can be made of any grain, the corn sensitive are also at risk.

[125] Often found in sauces, dressings, and ice cream, glycerides are made from both animal and vegetable fats or oils, corn included.

[126] "GDL" is a recently appearing additive in cured meats made of corn.

[127] A common thickener, which can be produced from bulk corn sugars.

171

If Someone is Sensitive to Corn (continued)

Other products that may contain corn include:	To maximize safety:
Emollient creams.	*Ask manufacturer for safe line to use.*
Toothpastes.	*Non-allergenic brands.*
Cosmetics.	*Ask manufacturer for safe line to use.*
Adhesives for envelopes, stamps and stickers.	*Use self-stick.*
Aspirin.	*Alternative pain relievers like ibuprofen or acetaminophen.*
Laxatives.	*Natural dietary laxatives or check with health food store.*
Common brand name vitamins.	*Allergen-free vitamins.*
Bath powders	*All-talc powders, ask manufacturer to ensure complete safety.*

If Someone is Sensitive to Soy[128]

⊘ AVOID	☑ USE instead
Hydrolyzed vegetable protein.[129]	*Vegetable proteins where source is known (wheat, corn, potato).*
Soy lecithin.[130]	*Avoid.*
Miso.[131]	*Avoid.*
Mono-diglyceride.[132]	*Check for exact source or avoid.*
Monosodium glutamate.[133]	*Ask manufacturer for source.*
Natto.[134]	*Avoid.*

---

[128] Those allergic to soybeans may also cross-react to certain foods, such as peanuts, green peas, chickpeas, lima beans, string beans, wheat flour, rye flour, and barley flour. So take this into account when using substitutions. All of the following soy information derived from: How to Live With an Allergy to Soy, by Roxanne Nelson, and from Soy Allergy, About.com.

[129] (HVP) is a protein obtained from any vegetable, including soy beans, that is a flavor enhancer that can be used in soups, broths, sauces, gravies, flavoring and spice blends, canned and frozen vegetables, meats and poultry.

[130] Lecithin is extracted from soybean oil and is used in foods that are high in fats and oils to promote stabilization, antioxidation, crystallization, and spattering control. It is used as an emulsifier in chocolate. Most infant formulas contain soy lecithin.

[131] Miso used to flavor soups, sauces, dressings, marinades and pâtés, is a rich, salty condiment made from soybeans and a grain such as rice.

[132] Another soy derivative is used for emulsion in many foods.

[133] MSG may contain hydrolyzed protein that is often made from soy.

[134] More easily digested than whole soybeans, is made of fermented and cooked whole soybeans.

172

If Someone is Sensitive to Soy[135] (continued)

⊘ AVOID	☑ USE instead
Natural flavors.[136]	Ask manufacturer for specific ingredients of natural flavors.
Soy cheese, a substitute for sour cream or cream cheese, is made from soy milk.	Regular cheeses, sour cream, or cream cheese.
Soy fiber (okara, soy bran, soy isolate).	Oat or other grain fiber.
Soy flour.[137]	Oat, wheat, rice, or other flours.
Soy grits.[138]	Corn grits.
Soy milk, and its derivatives like soy yogurt.	Regular milk, goats milk, etc. and their derivatives.
Soy meal and soy oil are used in a number of items, including inks, soaps, and cosmetics.	Ask manufacturer for specifics. Buy items made with alternative vegetable dyes and by-products.
Soy oil[139], if cold pressed. Otherwise believed to contain no protein.	100% pure canola, olive, peanut, safflower or other "ok" oils.
Soy protein[140], Soy sauces,[141] Tempeh,[142], Tofu.[143]	Avoid.
Vegetable oil.	Products where source is clearly identified, or ask manufacturer.

[135] Those allergic to soybeans may also cross-react to other foods in this family such as peanuts, green peas, chickpeas, lima beans, string beans, wheat flour, rye flour, and barley flour. So take this into account when using substitutions. All of the following soy information derived from: "How to Live With an Allergy to Soy", by Roxanne Nelson, and from Soy Allergy, About.com.

[136] May be a soy derivative.

[137] Soy flour is often used to give a protein boost to recipes. Whether natural, defatted, and lecithinated, it is made from finely ground roasted soybeans.

[138] Made from toasted coarsely cracked soybeans, is used as a flour substitute.

[139] Natural oil extracted from whole soybeans, is the most widely used oil in the United States, accounting for more than 75 percent of total vegetable fats and oils intake margarines, Crisco and other vegetable shortenings, prepared pasta sauces, Worcestershire sauce, salad dressings, mayonnaise, canned tuna, dry lemonade mix, and hot chocolate mix. Most commercial baked goods like breads, rolls, cakes, cookies, and crackers contain soy oil. Some prepackaged cereals are also made with soy oil.

[140] Can be labeled as soy protein concentrate, isolated soy protein, textured soy protein (TSP), and textured soy flour (TSF). Textured soy flour is widely used as meat extender. Most soup bouillons contain some form of soy protein. Many meat alternatives contain soy protein or tofu.

[141] Most common is Tamari (a by-product of making miso), Shoyu (a blend of soy beans and wheat), and Teriyaki (with added sugar, vinegar and spices), are dark brown liquids made from soy beans that have undergone a fermenting process.

[142] Traditional Indonesian food, a chunky, tender soybean cake.

[143] Also known as soybean curd, is a soft cheese-like food made by curdling fresh hot soymilk with a coagulant. It is a bland product that easily absorbs flavors of other ingredients. Can simulate various meats when mixed with other ingredients. Also, at press time a new form of soy is getting attention—edamame—which is fresh, green soybeans. Avoid, if soy-sensitive.

173

If Someone is Sensitive to Soy[144] (continued)

Vegetable protein.	*Products where source is clearly identified, or ask manufacturer.*
Vitamin E. [145]	*Cod Liver Oil for similar health benefits, or use soy-free Vitamin E .*

Summing it All Up

- The first step to being a good safe shopper for your food sensitive child is to be an *educated* shopper.

- *FDA labeling laws* have greatly improved our ability to see what's inside a package before we open it. But...

- *Vigilance* is still required for shopping trips because:
  - FDA laws exempt certain ingredients from being listed because of minimal nutritional impact
  - Small food manufacturers are exempt from labeling laws
  - Items used for "flavoring," "color", or as "spices"need not be individually listed.

- *You can* maximize your shopping trips if you:
  - *ALWAYS read the label,* even if you're familiar with the
  - product. Recipes change frequently and so do ingredients.
  - What's safe one time may not be the next.
  - *Contact the manufacturer* if you're not sure of ingredients.
  - Ask what is in a product, not what is NOT in a product.
  - *Beware of hidden allergens*
  - *Become familiar with substitute products.*
  - *Use a safe shopping guide, available through the Celiac Society of America, Tri-Counties Shopping Guide, or the Food Allergy Network (contact information in Appendix), and compile your own list of "safe" foods that you can use in conjunction with those lists.*

---

[144] Soy-allergic people may also cross-react to certain foods, such as peanuts, green peas, chick peas, lima beans, string beans, wheat flour, rye flour, and barley flour. Take this into account when using substitutions. Source: How to Live With an Allergy to Soy, by Roxanne Nelson, and from Soy Allergy, About.com.
[145] Contains soybean oil.

Chapter X
Kitchen Zen Revisited

So... now you know that your child is sensitive to a food or foods, you've learned all you can about it, know how to stay up to date on it, and have educated your child and everyone else about it as well.

Your child's health-esteem meter is off the charts. She's got the best health advocacy team anyone could want. You can plan menus, read labels, shop for groceries, and dine out with ease and efficiency (or at least you will with practice!). What's left? How about a little kitchen razzle-dazzle? Some tasty things to put in those menu plans, fresh from your own kitchen, made with love in a state of Zen-like, non-cross-contaminated grace!

The Basics
Cooking for the food-sensitive doesn't have to be hard, but it can be a little different from "traditional" cooking. Some of the substitutions for wheat flour, for instance, create different textures or flavors. Milk substitutions can also create different textures and flavors, depending on the type of substitute you use. You'll have to experiment a little and see what your family enjoys the most. I've found that most of the time, my family doesn't notice substitutions in recipes.

There are three basic substitutions you'll have to make for the food-sensitive diners in your home—wheat, milk, and eggs. Some families have to avoid just one of these ingredients; some have to avoid all three. Corn is easy to avoid if you don't use processed foods, so we only discuss it briefly here. Peanut, tree nuts, and shellfish are rarely an issue in most recipes. Soy can be a little harder to avoid because it isn't always listed as "soy" on the ingredient label. Instead, it hides behind words such as tofu, tempeh, or miso.

175

The following information on wheat, milk, and egg substitutes is reprinted with permission from cookbooks by Carol Fenster, Ph.D., Savory Palate, Inc.

Gluten-free Substitutions

If your child is sensitive to gluten, you need to avoid all gluten containing flours in your baking and cooking. These include—besides the obvious wheat flour—spelt, kamut, rye, barley, and oats.[146]

> "I make my own mayonnaise and salad dressings and make a lot of soups"
> —Lorraine

Non-gluten flours typically used as substitutes for wheat flour include the easily available rice flours (brown and white), soy, and corn. Baked items made with any one of these flours alone—especially the rice flours—tend to be grainy and heavy, but serviceable. Often, other "flours" are mixed in—such as tapioca flour, potato starch, arrowroot or cornstarch—to provide the necessary lightness in baked goods as well as elasticity and a crispy, browned exterior. In addition, bakers add an ingredient called xanthan gum or guar gum to prevent crumbling in baked goods.

Recently, the availability of other non-grain flours has helped improve gluten-free baking. For example, flours made from beans (garbanzo, Romano, or cranberry beans, and fava), sorghum (also called milo), quinoa, amaranth, and buckwheat greatly improve the quality, nutrition, and taste of non-wheat flour recipes, and are very versatile and easy to use. [147]

Combine these flours with others—such as tapioca, potato starch, or arrowroot—and you can recreate just about any traditional wheat flour recipe with impressive results. Other non-grain flours just beginning to gain wider acceptance

---

[146] From Food Allergy Organization. Oats are still off-limits to celiacs, but see footnotes 7 and 30 for more information about this controversial grain.

[147] See Gluten-Free Living newsletter, (May/June 1998) for an excellent discussion on the safety of these grains for the celiac diet.

include flours from chestnuts, almonds, peas, sweet potatoes, wild rice, and Indian rice grass (known as Montina).

You may be wondering how to successfully combine these strange new flours into something palatable. Well, if you don't consider yourself a baker—and many people don't—you'll be pleased to know that there are commercially prepared gluten-free flour mixes available in health food stores and some grocery stores. They work just like the flour mixes you bought before your family became gluten-free.

> *"Get creative! If you like to bread chicken and fry it, coat it in cornstarch and fry it! If you like croutons, deep fry some gluten-free bread."*—Danna

But if you want to make your own mixes, the following gluten-free mixes work well in just about any recipe, and particularly well in the recipes in Chapter 11.

Gluten-Free Flour Mixes*

Rice Flour Mix (#1)	Bean Flour Mix (#2)
3 cups brown rice flour	1 2/3 cups garbanzo/fava flour**
1 1/4 cups potato starch or cornstarch	2 cups potato starch or cornstarch
3/4 cup tapioca flour	2/3 cup tapioca flour
	2/3 cup sorghum flour
	**By Authentic Foods, Bob's Red Mill, or
*Mixes make 5 cups	Ener-G Foods.

As you become more experienced with these mixes, you'll learn to judge if the dough or batter is too dry, too moist, or just right. For best results, prepare the mixes ahead of time and store them in your refrigerator. Be sure to bring your mix to room temperature before measuring since cold flour measures differently.

You might also want to experiment with developing your own baking mixes with other acceptable flours such as quinoa, amaranth, or buckwheat. Use the charts on the following pages to help you, remembering that most mixes do better with a blend of higher-protein flours along with some "starchy" flours for lightness and better flavor.

Baking with Gluten-Free Flours

This table presents a summary of the baking characteristics and storage recommendations for wheat-free flours (and grains) used in this book.

FLOUR	CHARACTERISTICS
Arrowroot	Silky white powder from West Indies root. Good in baking because it adds no flavor of its own and lightens baked goods. Produces golden brown crust when used as breading. Replaces cornstarch or tapioca flour in baking.
Bean Flour	Two basic kinds of bean flour: (1) pure garbanzo or chickpea flour, and (2) blend of garbanzo and fava beans (by Authentic Foods, Bob's Red Mill, and Ener-G). Both flours are slightly yellow in color, provide beneficial protein for baking, and have a very slight "beany" taste. May totally replace rice flour in baking.
Corn Flour	Light yellow in color. Combine with other flours, including cornmeal, in baked goods. Refrigerate.
Corn meal	White or yellow (which has higher Vitamin A) with corn flavor. Excellent in corn bread, muffins, and waffles—especially when blended with corn flour.
Cornstarch	Snow-white, flavorless, and powdery. Lightens baked goods, but use only in combination with other flours. Commonly used as thickener in sauces and gravies.

Note: Ask your health professional if these alternatives are safe for your diet.

178

Baking with Gluten-Free Flours
(continued)

FLOUR	CHARACTERISTICS
Potato Flour	Heavy, light yellow flour made from whole potatoes. Use in very small quantities in baking; adds crispness and body to baked goods. Made from whole potatoes, including the skins. Strong potato flavor. Refrigerate.
Potato Starch	Very white, bland powder. Excellent baking properties when combined with others flours and eggs. Lumps easily; stir before measuring. Made from starch of potatoes. Not the same as potato flour, which is made from whole potatoes—including the skin.
Rice Flour White and Brown	White rice flour is white; nutritionally inferior. Brown rice flour is very light tan, but higher in nutrients. Bland, pleasant flavor. Dry and gritty alone; better if combined with other flours. Use as 2/3 of total flour mix. Outer layers are milled away to form rice bran and rice polish. Refrigerate brown rice flour, rice bran, and rice polish.
Sorghum	Light tan color, flavor similar to wheat—but can be bitter in large quantities. Somewhat dry, best used as no more than 15% of flour mix. Adds important protein to baked goods.
Soy	Light tan color. Bland, somewhat "nutty" flavor–almost bean-like. Excellent in baked goods with nuts, fruits, or chocolate. Best to combine with other flours such as rice and potato starch. Refrigerate due to higher fat/protein content.

Note: Ask your health professional if these alternatives are safe for your diet.

179

Baking with Gluten-Free Flours
(continued)

FLOUR	CHARACTERISTICS
Sweet Rice	White in color, bland flavor. Not the same as white rice flour. Best used as small portion of flour mix. Does not replace white or brown rice flour. Sometimes called sticky rice or glutinous rice—but contains no wheat gluten. "Stickiness" binds baked goods. Makes smooth, creamy sauces and gravies.
Tapioca	Snow-white, velvety powder with "anonymous" flavor. Made from cassava plant; use in place of arrowroot. Excellent in baked products as 25-50% of total flour. Lightens baked goods; adds "chewiness" to breads. Browns nicely; crispy breading.

"New" Flours for the Gluten-Free Diet

Amaranth	Light brown color. Nutty flavor. Good in baking; browns well. Use as 10-25% of total flour. Refrigerate.
Buckwheat	Choose lighter buckwheat flour from unroasted groats for lighter flavor. Combine with other flours (no more than 50%) for best results. Refrigerate.
Indian Rice Grass (Montina)	Light brown. Not commercially available yet. Great in baking, when mixed with other flours. Good flavor. Shelf-stable.
Millet	Light tan, high-protein, high-alkaline flour. Easy to digest. Best mixed with other flours. Becomes bitter and rancid quickly, so refrigerate or freeze.
Quinoa (keen-wah)	Light tan in color. Strong, nutty flavor can dominate so use as 10-15% of total flour. High-lysine protein content. Refrigerate.

Note: Ask your health professional if these alternatives are safe for your diet.

180

Substitutes for Wheat as Thickener
In place of 1 tablespoon of wheat flour, use:

INGREDIENT/ AMOUNT	TRAITS	SUGGESTED USES
Arrowroot – 1 1/2 tsp.	Mix with cold liquid before using. Thickens at lower temperature than wheat flour or cornstarch. Better for sauces that aren't boiled. Add during last 5 minutes of cooking. Serve immediately. Clear, shiny, semi-soft when cool.	Any food requiring clear, shiny sauce, but good for egg or starch dishes where high heat is undesirable. Gives appearance of oil even if none used.
Cornstarch – 1 1/2 tsp.	Mix with cold liquid before using. Stir just until boiling. Makes clear, shiny sauce. Rigid when cool.	Puddings, pie fillings, fruit sauces, soups. Gives appearance of oil if none used.
Kudzu (kuzu) Powder – 3/4 tsp.	Dissolve in cold water first. Odorless, tasteless. Makes smooth, transparent, soft sauces.	Puddings, pie fillings, and other dishes that must have "gelatin-like" consistency
Sweet Rice Flour – 1 tbsp.	Excellent thickening agent. Has no gluten.	Sauces such as vegetable sauces.
Rice Flour – 1 tbsp.	Mix with cold liquid before using. Somewhat grainy.	Soups, stews, or gravies or hearty, robust sauces
Tapioca Flour – 1 1/2 Tbsp.	Mix with cold or hot liquid first. Add during last 5 minutes of cooking. Clear, shiny sauce. Thick, soft gel when cool.	Soups, stews, gravies, potato dishes
Quick-Cooking Tapioca – 2 tsp.	Mix with fruit, let stand 15 minutes before baking.	Fruit pies, cobblers, and tapioca pudding
Xanthan Gum – 1 tsp.	Mix with dry ingredients first, then add to recipe.	Puddings, salad dressings, gravies

Note: Ask your health professional if these alternatives are safe for your diet.

Wheat Flour Equivalents

Use this table to convert your own recipes to gluten-free. Each flour has unique characteristics that affect the texture, taste, and look of baked goods—so use a blend of flours, not just one.

In place of 1 cup of wheat flour, use [148]:

FLOUR	AMOUNT
Amaranth	1 cup
Arrowroot	1 cup
Buckwheat	7/8 cup
Corn Flour	1 cup
Cornmeal	3/4 cup coarse grind 1 cup fine grind
Cornstarch	3/4 cup
Garbanzo (Chickpea) Flour	3/4 cup
Garfava Flour (Garbanzo/Chick-pea and Fava/Broad Bean Flour)	7/8 cup (use 1:1 ratio in dishes under 1 cup flour)
Indian Rice Grass (Montina)	1 cup
Millet	1 cup
Nuts (ground fine)	1/2 cup
Potato Starch or Potato Starch Flour	3/4 cup
Quinoa	1 cup
Rice Flour (Brown or White)	7/8 cup
Sorghum Flour (milo)	7/8 cup
Soy Flour	1/2 cup+1/2 cup potato starch.
Sweet Rice Flour	7/8 cup
Tapioca Flour or Tapioca Starch	1 cup

Gluten-Free Baking Tips

- Replace wheat flour with a mix of flours—not just one flour—to maximize the unique, important traits of each.
- Loosely spoon flour into measuring cup. Level top with knife. Don't "round" unless told to and never pack flour down.

---

[148] Variations in flour milling processes may affect consistency and texture of flours across different manufacturers. When you find a brand you like, stick with it.

- Use up to 25% more leavening (e.g., yeast). Boost flavor by adding 1/3 to 1/2 more spices or herbs to compensate for loss of wheat flavor.
- Use xanthan gum or guar gum to improve texture and reduce crumbling. A teaspoon of unflavored gelatin also helps reduce the grainy, crumbly texture of breads, muffins, and cookies.
- Gluten-free baked goods are heavier. An extra egg in baked goods adds moisture, improves texture, and adds protein, too.
- Use small, non-stick baking pans instead of one large one. Generously grease with safe shortening or oil before using. Use dry measure cups to measure dry ingredients; liquid measure cups for liquids.
- Invest in a bread machine, but be careful of cross-contamination if it's used for gluten and gluten-free bread. If programmable, carefully adjust settings until you get desired results. Food processors and heavy-duty mixers assure thorough mixing. Use non-stick cookie sheets or parchment paper, Teflon® sheets, or Silpat® liners to avoid sticking.

Baking with Milk Substitutes

Dairy products are among the easiest ingredients to make substitutions for in baking, although they lend subtle flavors and may affect browning of baked goods. Read labels to avoid problem ingredients such as casein or barley malt. Choose low-sugar versions for savory dishes.

SUBSTITUTE	AMOUNT	WHEN TO USE/TIPS
Rice Milk (rice beverage) Buy fortified brands.	1 cup. Mild flavor, white color.	Slightly sweet. Reduce by 2 Tbsp. per cup if buttermilk substitute. Check GF status.
Soy Milk (soy beverage) Buy fortified brands.	1 cup. Slight soy flavor, tan color.	Use herbs and seasonings to mask soy flavor. Darkens baked goods. Buy liquid or reconstitute powder.
Nut Milk (usually almond)	1 cup. Mild, nutty flavor. Light tan.	Best in desserts. Tastes a bit "off" in savory dishes. Nut-allergic should avoid.

NOTE: Ask your health professional if these alternatives are safe for your diet.

Baking with Milk Substitutes
*(*continued)

SUBSTITUTE	AMOUNT	WHEN TO USE/TIPS
Goat Milk or Powder	1 cup.	Not recommended for those with cow milk allergies or lactose intolerance. (Food Allergy Network newsletter, Vol. 5, #4, April-May, 1996)
Oat Milk	1 cup	Not for the gluten-sensitive.
Coconut Milk	1 cup	Very high in fat.

If the recipe calls for dry milk powder: Use same amount of non-dairy milk powder. Read labels to avoid problem ingredients such as casein. Or, omit dry milk powder and add same amount of sweet rice flour. Without dry milk powder, baked goods won't brown as nicely and yeast breads won't rise as much.

In place of 1 cup evaporated skim milk, use:

SUBSTITUTE	AMOUNT	WHEN TO USE/TIPS
Ener-G® NutQuik or SoyQuik or other non-dairy milk powder.	1 cup reconstituted at double strength.	Recipes using evaporated skim milk. Flavors will be stronger. Calories and nutrient values double.
Other non-dairy liquid	7/8 cup	Use potato water (from boiling potatoes) in bread recipes.

The suggestions offered in this section are primarily for baking. Bear in mind, however, that the same amount of milk substitute such as rice, soy, or nut milk can be used in non-baked items —such as milkshakes, puddings, ice cream, or smoothies.

In place of butter, use equal amounts of non-dairy margarine, spread, or vegetable oil of your choice—although sometimes the amount of oil will need to be reduced by 25%. In appropriate recipes, use equal amounts of bacon drippings or fat.

NOTE: Ask your health professional if these alternatives are safe for your diet.

In place of 1 cup buttermilk, use:

SUBSTITUTE	AMOUNT	WHEN TO USE/TIPS
Use 1-2 Tbsp. fresh lemon juice or cider vinegar and enough rice, soy, or nut milk to equal 1 cup.	1 cup.	Any recipe calling for buttermilk. Some non-dairy milks produce a thinner buttermilk. If so, use 2 tablespoons less of non-dairy buttermilk per cup specified in recipe.

Density of Milk: Whether you're using liquid non-dairy milks or mix your own from powder, remember that the thinner the milk the less you'll need. For example, reduce liquid by 1 tablespoon per cup if you use skim milk in place of whole milk, or very thin rice milk instead of a thicker version. You may need to experiment a bit to achieve the desired results since liquid milk densities vary by brand and the ratio of powder to water will affect the density of milks made from non-dairy powders.

Also, when rice milk is used in a recipe that will be thickened, such as pudding, add 2 teaspoons unflavored gelatin powder dissolved in 1/4 cup of the recipe liquid for 10 minutes. This improves the thickening process.

Note that plain milk may contain one set of ingredients but flavored versions may contain different ingredients.

Lactose-Reduced Milk: You may use lactose-reduced milk in these recipes. However, make sure you can tolerate these milks and be certain to read the label to make sure they contain no other offending ingredients.

Cheese: Although there are several "non-dairy" cheeses such as Parmesan cheese made from rice, soy, or nuts, it is difficult to find one that doesn't have additional problem ingredients. Some for example, may contain the milk proteins calcium caseinate,

Note: Ask your health professional if these alternatives are safe for your diet.

185

sodium caseinate, or casein. Others include oats, which celiacs should avoid, or texturized vegetable protein, which can come from a variety of sources, but is often soy.

Sour Cream and Cream Cheese: Soyco® makes rice-based sour cream and cream cheese, but check the label to make sure it's right for your diet and be aware that casein is present in both items. Soymage® makes a casein-free sour cream alternative. You may use the same amount of mayonnaise in place of sour cream or cream cheese—in appropriate recipes. Keep in touch with your natural food store. New, non-dairy cheeses are being developed.

In place of 1 cup yogurt, use:

SUBSTITUTE	AMOUNT	WHEN TO USE/TIPS
Goat Yogurt	1 cup	Not recommended for those with cow milk allergy and lactose intolerance.
Soy Yogurt	1 cup	Doesn't heat well, but good for dips, ice cream. Won't drain.
Non-Dairy Milk Liquid	2/3 cup	Any recipe with yogurt. Add in 1/3 cup increments, to avoid adding too much.

Note: Ask your health professional if these alternatives are safe for your diet.

Baking with Egg Substitutes

Eggs are one of the hardest ingredients to exclude because they play such critical roles in baking. For example, they can be used as binding agents (hold ingredients together), moisturizers (add moisture), or as leavening agents (make things rise) in baking.

It's good to have some understanding of these different purposes, so you can use appropriate substitutes to get the best results. Remember—compared to their egg-laden counterparts, egg-free baked goods don't rise as much and are denser.

Eggs As Binders:
If the recipe has only one egg but contains a fair amount of baking powder or baking soda, then the egg is the binder.

In place of 1 egg as a binder, use:

SUBSTITUTE	AMOUNT	WHEN TO USE/TIPS
Tofu (soft silken) by Mori-Nu®	1/4 cup for each egg.	Cakes, cookies, breads. Baked goods won't brown as much and are moist and heavy. Blend with recipe liquid first until smooth.
Unflavored Gelatin - (Knox brand) or agar	Mix 1 envelope gelatin in 1 cup boiling water. 1 large egg = 3 Tbsp. gelatin	Baked goods that don't need to rise much like cookies, bars, flatbreads. Flavorless. Refrigerate. Microwave to liquefy after refrigeration.
Flaxseed (Available as brown or golden seeds or as ground flaxmeal. If using flaxseeds, first pulverize to powder consistency in coffee grinder.)	Soak 1 tsp. flaxmeal in 1/3 cup boiling water for 5 min. 1 egg (large) =1/4 cup flax mix	Best in cookies, bars. Cool before using. Best in "dark" color dishes. Mild flavor. Baked goods are heavy, dense. Slight laxative effect. Refrigerate to avoid rancidity. Bake dish slightly longer; 25° lower. Reduce oil 1 to 2 Tbsp

Note: Ask your health professional if these alternatives are safe for your diet.

Liquid Egg Substitutes: *People with egg allergies cannot safely consume these products because they still contain eggs*! The yolks have been removed to reduce the fat and cholesterol, but the whites remain. Also, some egg substitutes contain other problem ingredients such as modified food starch—which may or may not be wheat-based. Read the label.

Eggs as Leavening Agents:
If there are no other ingredients that make the baked item rise (such as baking powder), then the egg is the leavening agent.

In place of 1 egg as a leavener, use:

SUBSTITUTE	AMOUNT	WHEN TO USE/TIPS
Ener-G ® Egg Replacer (potato starch, tapioca, calcium lactate, calcium carbonate, citric acid, carbohydrate gum) Contains no dairy.	2-3 times more than manufacturer says.	All baked goods. Flavorless; won't affect taste of recipe. For added lightness, whip in food processor or blender for 30 seconds.
Buttermilk-Soda	Replace all liquid with same amount buttermilk. Replace baking powder with same amount of baking soda, not exceeding 1 tsp. per cup of flour.	All baked goods, but this technique works best in dishes that don't require a lot of "rising" to look good, such as cookies, bars and flatbreads.
Carbonated Water	2 Tbsp. carbonated water and 2 tsp. flour	Best in bars and cookies that don't require much rising.

Note: Ask your health professional if these alternatives are safe for your diet.

188

Other Hints When Omitting Eggs As Leavening Agents

(1) Cream the fat and sweetener together with your electric mixer to add air and lightness. Then add dry ingredients.

(2) Whip the liquid ingredients in a food processor or blender for 30 seconds as another way of incorporating air into recipes.

(3) Add an extra 1/2 teaspoon baking powder per egg in baked goods. Do not exceed 1 teaspoon baking powder per cup of flour or a bitter taste will develop.

(4) Recipes with acidic liquids such as buttermilk, molasses, lemon juice, or vinegar tend to rise better than those with non-acidic liquids such as water or milk.

Eggs as Moisture
If there are leavening agents in the recipe such as baking powder, but not much other liquid, then the egg's purpose in a recipe is to add moisture.

Generally speaking, baked goods without eggs are somewhat heavier and denser than those with eggs. For that reason, slightly increase the leavening agent in egg-free recipes to compensate for the egg's natural leavening effect. In addition, using liquid sweeteners such as honey or molasses for part of the sugar in a recipe helps compensate for the loss of the "binding" effect of eggs.

In place of 1 egg as a moisturizer, use:

SUBSTITUTE	AMOUNT	WHEN TO USE/TIPS
Fruit juice, milk, or water	2 Tbsp. Increase leavening 25-50%.	Baked goods such as cakes, cookies, bars. May need to bake items slightly longer.

Note: Ask your health professional if these alternatives are safe for your diet.

189

In place of 1 egg as a moisturizer, use: (continued)

SUBSTITUTE	AMOUNT	WHEN TO USE/TIPS
Puréed fruit: Bananas, applesauce, apricots, pears, prunes. (The natural pectin in fruits, especially prunes, traps air which helps "lighten" baked goods.)	Use 1/4 cup. Increase leavening agent by 25-50%. May need to bake items slightly longer.	Baked goods where the fruit's flavor complements the overall dish such as applesauce in spice cakes, bananas in banana bread, apricots and pears in mild-flavored items, and prunes in dark, heavily-flavored items such as chocolate or spice cakes.

Corn-Free Substitutions

Unless you're preparing a specifically corn-based dish that contains corn meal or corn flour—which is unlikely if your child is sensitive to corn—the most common place you'll encounter corn in a recipe is through cornstarch or baking powder and you can replace both easily.

Replace	With
Cornstarch	Baking: An equal amount of potato starch or arrowroot. Thickening: See Wheat-Flour Equivalents on page 182.
Baking Powder (1 tsp). (Featherweight brand is corn-free)	Mixture of 1 tsp. cream of tartar, 1 tsp. arrowroot, and 1/2 tsp. baking soda, OR 3/4 tsp. baking soda plus 1 7/8 tsp. cream of tartar

Note: Ask your health professional if these alternatives are safe for your diet.

Cooking Up Something Good—Safely

The recipes in the next chapter represent a rather eclectic collection of relatively quick, easy, and tasty meals, snacks, and desserts that require a minimum of skill to prepare and cook.

I can't stress enough, though, that you need to be a tidy chef. The easiest thing to do is fix the same, safe meal for everyone. But if you're making some slightly different meals and side dishes—and some of those meals and side dishes have forbidden ingredients for your child—then be careful.

- *Keep counters clean* between preparations of food for non-food sensitive members of the family and meals for your food-sensitive child.

- *Don't use the same utensils* to prepare an allergen-free meal that you use for a regular meal—that includes things as seemingly benign as stirring a regular pot of pasta with the same spoon or fork you use to stir your child's gluten-free pasta.

- *Beware of other cross-contamination issues* from toasters, ovens, containers, pots, and pans.

- *Wash your hands frequently* and be careful when you're working in the kitchen. You can't munch on peanuts while preparing a meal for your peanut-sensitive child, or get croutons in your gluten-intolerant child's salad.

- *Keep other people's hands out of the food.* If family and friends want samples, give them separate "tasting" bowls to enjoy. That reduces the chances that someone might inadvertently contaminate your child's food.

- *Keep your mind on your work.* Remember your kitchen Zen and keep it holy. Focus on what you're doing instead of trying to do a dozen things at once. It's easy to grab the wrong ingredient if you're hurrying and not paying attention.

-191

Dietary Exchanges

The lists of substitutions we've just looked at comprise a type of exchange list, showing you how to exchange prohibited ingredients in recipes for safe ones. The same principal applies to overall meal preparation, to

"Keep it simple, at least at first. I have a large number of minimal preparation, throw-it-in-the-oven type meals already pre-planned for hectic work and Cub Scout days."—Lee

the foods you'll choose as side dishes and to prepare in different types of recipes.

The Diabetic Exchange list, typically used by diabetics to maximize nutrition, provides an excellent resource for helping you find safe equivalents for your food-sensitive child. In this list, foods are grouped together by type, with each serving having approximately the same amount of carbohydrate, protein, fat, and calories as any of the other foods on the list. One "exchange" or food on the list can be exchanged or traded evenly for any other item on the same list.

As you learn what foods you can exchange for others to meet recommended daily values in various food groups, you'll find that cooking and shopping becomes even easier. And, if your child learns how to make the proper exchanges early on, choosing safe and healthy foods becomes second nature for all of you.

Here's an example of fruit exchanges worth 15 grams of carbohydrate and 60 calories each.[149] Each item in the chart is exactly equal, in serving sizes given, to any other item in the chart.[150]

Apple, unpeeled, small 1 (4 oz)	Orange, small 1 (6.5 oz)
Banana, small 1 (4 oz)	Pear, large, fresh 1/2 (4oz)
Grapes, small 17 (3 oz)	Strawberries, whole 1 1/4 cups

---

[149] American Diabetes Association
[150] More extensive charts are available online from the American Diabetes Association, the USDA, and from other organizations. Another organization, Meals For You, offers a free, interactive database of recipes and menu plans with searchable dietary exchange charts. Information is available in the resource section of this book.

If your child can't have milk or dairy products, the ADA guidelines suggest exchanging one-cup of soy or rice milk (fortified) or kefir for one cup of whole milk. And the following starchy vegetables can be exchanged for one another (a serving of each item equals 15 grams of carbohydrate, three grams of protein, about 1 gram of fat, and provides 80 calories).

Corn 1/2 cup	Potato, mashed 1/2 cup
Green peas 1/2 cup	Squash, (e.g., acorn) 1/2 cup

Clearly, you don't need to be this precise when exchanging a forbidden food for a safe one, but the principal is the same. And, when you look at an exchange list, you get a very vivid picture of just how rich and varied a diet can be, and it should help you understand that removing one food or even a few foods from your child's diet won't bring the food pyramid tumbling down!

The Possibilities are Endless!

As you can see, we've come a long way from the initially gloomy diagnosis of food sensitivity in your child. What may have seemed like a sentence of a limited diet for life, should now appear as what it is: a world of dietary possibilities and choices that would have gone largely unnoticed if you thought your child could eat all the bread, milk, cheese, and eggs he wanted, along with all the other ingredients that go with the convenience foods we've grown to rely upon.

Your child's food sensitivities can, indeed, be limiting. Or his unique dietary requirements can broaden his culinary horizons and improve his health beyond anything most people ever even consider for themselves. The choice is yours...and your choices are literally endless!

Summing it All Up

- *Cooking for the food sensitive doesn't have to be hard,* but it can be a little different from "traditional" cooking. You can learn to use appropriate substitutions. With practice, you'll learn how those substitutions may affect texture and taste.

- *Cooking Up Good Things Safely.*

  - *Keep counters clean*
  - *Don't use the same utensils* to prepare allergen-free meals that you use for regular meals
  - *Beware of other cross-contamination issues* from toasters, ovens, containers, pots, and pans.
  - *Wash your hands frequently*
  - *Keep other people's hands out of the food*
  - *Keep your mind on your work*

- *Dietary Exchanges* are a good way to manage a food-sensitive diet, and can help you identify which foods to substitute for forbidden ones.

- *The possibilities are endless!* Instead of being limiting, realize that your child's food sensitivities open up a world of healthy dietary possibilities for your child and for the entire family!

Chapter XI
Ready, Set, Cook!

Wondering about this new lifestyle? Rest assured, allergen-free cooking is basically the same as any other cooking from scratch. You just change the ingredients to suit your needs.

The basic set of recipes here will help you get started. Follow them exactly the first time and if you make changes later, write everything down as you go. Soon you'll have your own unique, safe collection of recipes that everyone can enjoy.

The recipes are listed by category (e.g., breakfast or desserts) and labeled as G=gluten-free; D=dairy-free (lactose, whey, and casein-free); E=egg-free; N=nut-free; and S=soy-free. Recipes are also corn-free (C), but choose corn-free baking powder (e.g., Feath-erweight) and note that Kingsmill egg replacer contains corn. Instead of corn-based xanthan gum, use half again as much guar gum. See page 232 for additional tips.

The gluten-free flour mixes in Chapter 10 produce delicious results every time, whether you use the bean or rice flour mix. Persons with sensitivities to legumes should use the rice flour mix. Offending ingredients are omitted—or appropriate substitutes are given—in each recipe. If you can eat dairy products, use them in the same amount as the non-dairy substitutes. It is possible that some recipes will not be appropriate for your diet.

Even if you're a novice in the kitchen, these recipes are fail-proof. They are nutritious*, tasty, and kid-tested and approved. (A few are even kid-created!) So happy, allergen-free cooking! And don't forget to let your food-sensitive child help you out!

*Nutrient values for each recipe are derived from MasterCook, a software program that is briefly discussed (along with other software) in Chapter 8. Nutrient values are approximate and given for the base recipe only. When substitute ingredients are given, values are for the first one listed. For additional recipes, visit www.savorypalate.com.

195

Snacks

No child's day is complete without a snack or two (or three or four, sometimes!). Your food-sensitive child won't be excluded at snack time if you have these healthy treats on hand.*

Ants on a Log
Choose ingredients that are safe for your diet

Celery stalks (rinsed, dried)

Filling (choose for your diet)
   Peanut butter or soy butter
   Almond or cashew butter
   Cream cheese or goat cheese
   Hummus or guacamole

Ants (choose for your diet)
   Raisins or currants
   Dried sweetened cranberries
   Dried blueberries
   Walnuts, almonds, or pecans
   Sunflower or pumpkin seeds

Cut stalks (logs) into halves or thirds, crosswise. Fill hollow of each celery stalk with filling; top with "ants" of choice. One celery stalk serves 3.
Nutrient values vary depending on ingredients used.

Apples à la Mode
C, D (check sorbet), E, G, N (use seeds), S

4 large apples, cored
Frozen sorbet
Honey or agave nectar

Walnuts or seeds from sun-
   flowers or pumpkins

Place apples on lightly greased cookie sheet and bake in 325° oven until soft (about 10-15 minutes). Fill center with sorbet (or ice cream, if appropriate for your diet). Top with honey, nuts (or seeds). Serves 4.
Calories 237; Fat 3g; Protein 1g; Carb 56g; Chol 0mg; Sodium 3mg; Fiber 6g.

*For more snack ideas, see Carol Fenster's three cookbooks (in Bibliography).

196

Banana Pops
C, D, E, G, N, S

1 banana (ripe, firm)   2 wooden craft sticks
Toppings (choose for your diet)
Roll in honey, agave nectar, or melted dairy-free, soy-free
chocolate. Sprinkle with crushed nuts or sunflower/pumpkin
seeds, shredded coconut, sesame seeds, etc.

Peel and cut banana in half, crosswise. Insert wooden stick in
each half, lengthwise. Wrap in plastic and freeze. Remove
plastic wrap and dip in honey, agave nectar, or melted chocolate. Sprinkle with your favorite topping. Serves 2.
Nutrient values vary depending on ingredients used.

Beetle Bites
C, D, E, G, N, S

3 medium pears   Any of the following:
                                   apples, carrots, oranges,
                                   raisins, or currants

Cut pears in half for beetle body. Place skin side up on plate.
Use orange sections for wings, apple or carrot strips for anten-
nae and legs, and raisins for eyes and spots on body. Use addi-
tional carrot or apple strips as desired for additional details.
Serve on lettuce leaves, arranged on individual plates. Serves 6.
Nutrient values vary depending on ingredients used.

Party Mix
D, E, G, N (if no nuts in candy),

5 cups popcorn (popped)   1 cup candy corn or other
M&M's® (6 oz. package)   appropriate candy

Mix and serve. Makes 6 cups.
Nutrient values vary depending on ingredients used.

197

Traditional Crisp Rice Treats
D, E, G, N, S (check margarine for dairy or soy)

1/4 cup margarine or canola oil
5 cups small marshmallows
  (Jet-Puffed® is gluten-free)
6 cups crisp rice cereal (e.g., Barbara's®)
1/8 teaspoon salt (optional)

Melt margarine and marshmallows in large pan over low heat, stirring until completely melted. Remove from heat and add rice cereal, stirring until well coated. Press mixture into greased 13x9-inch dish. Cut into squares when cool. Serves 16.
Calories 115; Fat 3g; Protein 1g; Carb 19g, Chol 0mg; Sodium 83 mg; Fiber 1g.

Cinnamon Apple Rings
by T.M. Willingham
C, D, E, G, N, S (check sorbet)

4 to 5 Granny Smith apples
1/4 cup apple juice
1 teaspoon lemon juice
1/4 teaspoon cinnamon
1/8 teaspoon ground nutmeg
Frozen sorbet (optional)

Core, (peel, if desired), and thinly slice apples. Layer in 9-inch glass baking dish. Pour juices over apples. Sprinkle with cinnamon and nutmeg. Cover and microwave 5-7 minutes on high. Serve hot or cold. Top with frozen sorbet. Serves 6.
Calories 54; Fat 1g; Protein 1g; Carb 15g; Chol 0mg; Sodium 2mg; Fiber 2g.

Roasted Pumpkin Seeds
C, D, E, G, N, S

2 cups pumpkin seeds (shelled)   1 teaspoon canola oil

Combine seeds and oil in large bowl and stir till well coated. Spread seeds on cookie sheet and bake at 300° for 20 minutes, turning seeds every five minutes with spatula. Salt lightly. Cool. Serves 8.
Calories 195; Fat 17g; Protein 8g; Carb 6g; Chol 0mg; Sodium 6mg; Fiber 1g.

Fruit Kebabs
C, D, E, G, N, S

Grapes   **Strawberries**
Pineapple chunks   **Other fruits of choice**

Thread fruits onto 6-inch wooden skewer and serve with honey almond dip (below). The fruit kebabs can also be lightly grilled.

Salad Kebabs: Skewer pieces of cucumber, cherry tomatoes, sweet peppers, etc. Serve with salad dressing (see page 230).
Nutrient values depend on ingredients used.

Honey Almond Dip for Fruit
C (check yogurt ingredients), D (if using soy yogurt) E, G, N (if you use sunflower seeds), S (if using cow milk yogurt)

Plain, dairy-free yogurt or tofu   **3 tablespoons slivered almonds**
2 1/2 tablespoons honey   **or sunflower seeds**

Mix together and serve with assorted fruits. Serves 4.
Calories 120; Fat 6g; Protein 4g; Carb 14g; Chol 0mg; Sodium 5 mg; Fiber 1g.

Melon Bowls
C, D, E, G, N, S

2 medium cantaloupe   **1 cup strawberries, grapes, or**
                                    other small fruit, sliced

Cut cantaloupe in quarters. Scoop out seeds and fill center of each quarter with sliced fruit. Serve chilled. Serves 4.
Calories 110; Fat 1g; Protein 2g; Carb 27g; Chol 0mg; Sodium 50 mg; Fiber 3g.

Spiced Nuts
C, D, E, G, P, S
(Make sure pecans or walnuts are safe for your diet)

2 tablespoons canola oil
2 cups pecans or walnuts
1 teaspoon grated orange peel

1 teaspoon cinnamon
1/2 teaspoon nutmeg
1/4 teaspoon ginger

Toss nuts with oil. Mix remaining ingredients together and shake with nuts in resealable plastic bag until nuts are thoroughly coated. Spread in single layer on ungreased baking sheet. Bake at 300° for 20 minutes or until golden. Serves 8.
Calories 200; Fat 21g; Protein 2g; Carb 4g; Chol 0mg; Sodium 1mg; Fiber 2g

"Hot" Spiced Nuts: Coat nuts with 2 tablespoons olive oil, then mix with 1/4 teaspoon cayenne pepper and a dash of Tabasco® (or to taste). Bake at 300° on heavy baking sheet in single layer until crisp—about 15 minutes.

Orange Nuts: Coat nuts with boiled mixture of 1/4 cup sugar, 2 tablespoons orange juice, and 2 teaspoons grated orange peel. Spread coated nuts on waxed paper; cool completely.

Garbanzo Bean Nuts: Combine 1 teaspoon chili powder, 1/4 teaspoon ground cumin, 1/2 teaspoon garlic powder, and 1/2 teaspoon salt. Toss 1 can (16 oz.) drained garbanzo beans with 2 teaspoons olive oil. Then toss with spice mixture to coat thoroughly. Bake on large baking sheet for about 1 hour, shaking pan occasionally to promote even browning. Store in airtight container. Serves 8 (1/4 cup each).
Calories 200, Fat 4g, Protein, 10 g; Carb 30g; Chol 0mg; Sodium 150mg, Fiber 9g

Savory Crackers

By Carol Fenster, Ph.D. – *Special Diet Celebrations*, 1999
C, D (without Parmesan), E, G, N, S

1/2 cup Mix #1 or #2 (page 177)
1/4 cup sweet rice flour
1/2 teaspoon xanthan gum
1/4 teaspoon baking soda
1/2 teaspoon salt
2 tablespoons non-dairy
   Parmesan cheese (or sweet
   rice flour)

1 teaspoon grated fresh onion
2 tablespoons canola oil
1 tablespoon honey
3 tablespoons toasted sesame seeds
2 tablespoons soy or rice milk
1 teaspoon cider vinegar

Preheat oven to 350°. Grease baking sheet or use parchment paper.

In food processor, combine flours, xanthan gum, baking soda, salt, Parmesan cheese, and onion. Add oil, honey, and sesame seeds and pulse until dough resembles coarse crumbs. Add milk and vinegar and process until dough forms soft ball.

Shape dough into 20 balls, each 1-inch in diameter, and place on baking sheet at least 2 inches apart. Using bottom of drinking glass or a rolling pin, flatten balls to approximately 1/8-inch thick. Use your fingers to smooth edges of circle. (Or, roll dough to 1/8-inch thickness on cookie sheet. Then, cut cookies to desired shapes with cookie cutters. Peel off unused dough and hand shape these scraps into crackers.)

Bake for 12-15 minutes, or until crackers look firm and slightly toasted. Turn each cracker and bake another 5-7 minutes or until golden brown. (Sprinkle with additional sesame seeds and salt, if desired). Makes about 20 crackers. Serves 10 (2 crackers each).

Calories 115; Fat 5g, Protein 2g, Carb 17g, Chol 1mg, Sodium 160mg, Fiber 1g

201

Hummus (Chickpea Pate)
by Kaylene Irwin
C, D, E, G, N, S

2 cups chickpeas (garbanzo
   beans), cooked (reserve juice)
1/2 clove garlic, minced
1/4 cup Tahini or 1 finely
   grated carrot

2 tablespoons lemon juice
1/4 teaspoon salt
1 tablespoon chopped parsley
1/4 teaspoon ground cumin
1/4 teaspoon paprika

Combine all ingredients in food processor and blend. Add small amounts of reserved chickpea juice, if needed, to achieve desired consistency. Serves 8.

Calories 250; Fat 7g; Protein 11g; Carb 33g; Chol 0mg; Sodium 80mg; Fiber 9g

Salsa
by Melissa Taylor, FAST
C, D, E, G, N, S (check tomato paste)

1 cup water
1 can (4.5 oz) green chiles
1 teaspoon sugar
1 teaspoon lemon juice
3/4 cup tomato paste

1/4 cup chopped jalapeños*
1 tablespoon cider vinegar
1 teaspoon xanthan gum
1/8 teaspoon salt
1/8 teaspoon onion powder

Combine all ingredients in food processor or blender and whirl to desired consistency. Transfer to container and store in freezer. Serves 8.

*Melissa recommends pickled jalapeños sold in a jar. Put 1/4 cup in food processor with all the juice that is in the jar.

Calories 29; Fat 1g Protein 1g; Carb 7g; Chol 0mg; Sodium 51mg; Fiber 1g

Fruit Pops
adapted from a recipe by Lorraine Rendon
C, D, E, G, N, S (use rice milk)

1 cup soy or rice milk
1 banana

1/2 pint strawberries or fruit
      of choice
Wooden craft sticks (flat)

Blend milk, banana, and strawberries in blender. Add additional fruit or crushed ice for desired consistency. Pour into four small plastic cups. Insert stick and freeze. Serves 4.

Or, instead of freezing, pour into cups and serve as a shake.

Calories 65; Fat 2g; Protein 2g; Carb 10g; Chol 0mg; Sodium 30mg; Fiber 1g

Wormy Wiggler
C, D (check candy), E, G, N, S

8 oz. (1 pkg.) orange-flavored
    gelatin*

Pure fruit leather cut into
worm shapes

*Note: If food coloring is a problem, use unflavored gelatin and replace water with orange juice.

Prepare gelatin according to package directions. Pour into 9-inch pie plate (coated with cooking spray for easier removal). Refrigerate for 90 minutes, or until partly thickened. Press gummy worms into gelatin. Refrigerate another 2 hours until firm. To unmold, dip pie plate bottom in warm water for about 15 seconds, then gently loosen gelatin by running sharp knife around edges. Place moistened dish over center of pie plate, then invert. Decorate with additional worms. Serves 8.

Calories 108; Fat 0g; Protein 10g; Carb 17g; Chol 0mg; Sodium 49mg; Fiber 0mg

Good Morning!

Make sure your family gets off to a nutritious start with these delicious breakfast ideas.*

Granola Bars

C, D, E, G, N (if you use sunflower or sesame seed butter), S

1 cup honey	6 cups Pacific Grain® Nutty
1 cup peanut butter*	rice cereal
1 cup almonds**	1/2 cup dairy-free, soy-free
1/2 cup chopped dates	chocolate chips

Melt honey and peanut butter together; mix with remaining ingredients. Press into greased baking 9 x 13-inch. Cut into 16 squares or bars when cooled. Serves 16.

*Or butters made from almond, cashew, sunflower, or sesame (Tahini).
**Or sunflower or pumpkin seeds.
Calories 325; Fat 12g; Protein 7g; Carb 50g; Chol 0mg; Sodium 130mg; Fiber 3g

Waffles

By Carol Fenster, Ph.D. – *Special Diet Celebrations*, 1999
C, D, E, N, S

1 3/4 cups Mix # 1 or #2 (page 177)	2 tablespoons canola oil
2 teaspoons baking powder**	2 tablespoons cider vinegar
1/2 teaspoon salt	1 1/3 cups soy or rice milk
1 tablespoon sugar	1 teaspoon vanilla extract
2 large eggs or 1/2 cup soft	
silken tofu or flax mix***	**Featherweight brand
	***See page 231

Combine dry ingredients (flour through sugar) in medium bowl. In separate bowl, whisk together eggs (or tofu or flax), oil, vinegar, milk, and vanilla until completely smooth. Whisk liquids into flour just until combined. Cook on waffle iron, according to manufacturer instructions. Makes 6.
Calories 330; Fat 8g, Protein 6g, Carb 60g, Chol 60mg, Sod 320mg, Fiber 3g

*For more breakfast recipes, see Carol Fenster's three cookbooks (in Bibliography).

Rice Flour Pancakes
by T.M. Willingham
C, D, E (use water), G, N, S (use rice milk)

2 cups Mix #1 (page 177)	1 3/4 cups soy or rice milk
4 teaspoons baking powder*	1 egg, beaten or 1/4 cup water
2 teaspoons sugar	1 tablespoon canola oil
1 teaspoon salt	1 teaspoon vanilla extract
1/4 teaspoon baking soda	1/2 teaspoon xanthan gum

*Featherweight brand

Heat griddle or pan to 375° (or until water droplets dance on surface). In a pitcher or tall container, whisk together flour, baking powder, salt, and sugar. Add milk, egg, oil, and vanilla and whisk until just blended. Pour on griddle to form 2 to 4-inch pancakes. Turn with spatula when edges turn shiny and bottom browns (lift slightly with spatula to check underside). Cook other side about half as long. Serve with maple syrup. Makes 12 to 18 pancakes. Serves 6.

Calories 240; Fat 5g; Protein 5g; Carb 45g; Chol 30mg; Sodium 650mg; Fiber 3g.

French Toast
by T.M. Willingham
C, D, G, N, S (use rice milk)

8 slices gluten-free bread	1/2 cup soy or rice milk
2 eggs, beaten	1 tablespoon canola oil

Stir together eggs and milk. Soak bread in mixture and fry in non-stick skillet until golden on both sides. (If bread is hard or stale, microwave for few seconds first.) Serves 4.

Calories 235; Fat 8g; Protein 8g; Carb 25g, Chol 91mg; Sodium 300mg; Fiber 2g.

Egg-Free French Toast: Soak 8 slices of bread 1 cup non-dairy milk and 1/4 cup pure maple syrup. In nonstick skillet, fry on both sides in 1 tablespoon canola oil until golden.

Calories 225; Fat 6g; Protein 5g; Carb 38g; Chol 1mg; Sodium 270mg; Fiber 2g.

French Toast Sticks: Follow above procedures, but cut each bread slice into 4 strips before proceeding.

Hash Brown Egg Casserole
by T.M. Willingham
C, D, G, N, S

1 onion, chopped	1 red bell pepper, chopped
1 tablespoon canola oil	8 eggs, slightly beaten
2 small potatoes (peeled, cubed)	1/4 teaspoon salt
1 green pepper, chopped	1/8 teaspoon black pepper

Sauté onions in oil in non-stick pan until soft. Add potatoes and fry, stirring often, until they start to brown. Add peppers and eggs. Cook, stirring constantly, until eggs are set. Season with salt and pepper. Serves 6.

Calories 138; Fat 8g; Protein 8g; Carb 8g; Chol 240 mg; Sodium 250; Fiber 1g

Biscuits
by Carol Fenster, Ph.D. – *Special Diet Solutions*, 1999
C, D, E, G, N

1/4 cup margarine or spread	3/4 teaspoon baking soda
2/3 cup soy or rice milk	1 teaspoon xanthan gum
1 3/4 cups Mix #1 or #2 (page 177)	1/2 teaspoon salt
1 1/2 teaspoons cream of tartar	1 teaspoon sugar

Preheat oven to 400°. Line baking sheet with parchment paper or grease generously. Set aside.

Place all ingredients in food processor and pulse just until mixed. Working quickly, drop 8 balls of dough on baking sheet (an ice cream scoop works great for this). Bake for 15 minutes or until browned. Serves 8.

Calories 180; Fat 8g, Prot. 2g, Carb. 30g, Chol. 0mg, Sodium 300mg, Fiber 1g

Apricot-Honey Butter: by Kathy Lundquist, C, D, E, G, N
Combine 1/2 cup butter or dairy-free margarine, softened, with 1/2 cup apricot preserves, and 4 tablespoons honey. Serve with biscuits, waffles, etc. Serves 8.

Calories per tablespoon 180; Fat 11g; Protein 1g; Carb 22g; Chol 0mg; Sodium 140; Fiber 1g

Basic Muffins
by Carol Fenster, Ph.D. – *Special Diet Solutions*, 1998
C, D, E, G, N, S (without soy milk and tofu)

Dry Ingredients	Liquid Ingredients
2 1/3 cups Mix #1 or #2 (page 177)	1 cup soy or rice milk
1 teaspoon xanthan gum	1/4 cup canola oil
1 teaspoon unflavored gelatin	2 large eggs or 1/2 cup silken
2 1/2 teaspoons baking powder*	tofu or 1/2 cup flax mix (page 231)
1/2 cup sugar	1 teaspoon vanilla extract
1 teaspoon salt	1 tablespoon grated lemon peel
*Featherweight brand	

Preheat oven to 375°. Grease standard 12-cup, non-stick muffin tin or use paper liners.

Combine dry ingredients. Make well in center.

In another bowl, whisk together liquid ingredients until very smooth. Pour into well of flour mixture. Stir just until ingredients are moistened.

Transfer batter to prepared pans. Bake 20-25 minutes—or until tops of muffins are lightly browned. Remove from oven. Cool. Serves 12.

Calories 200, Fat 6g, Prot. 3g, Carb. 34g, Chol. 36 mg, Sodium 266 mg, Fiber 1 g

Banana Chocolate Chip Muffins: Add 1 cup mashed, ripe bananas and 1 teaspoon ground cinnamon to batter. After batter is mixed, stir in 1 cup semi-sweet chocolate chips (choose dairy-free, gluten-free, soy-free version)

Blueberry Lemon Muffins: Fold in 1 cup fresh blueberries.

Cranberry Orange Muffins: Fold in 1 cup finely chopped fresh cranberries or Craisins® and 1 tablespoon grated orange peel.

Lemon Craisin® Muffins: Increase grated lemon peel to 2 tablespoons and add 1 cup Craisins®.

Lemon-Poppy Seed Muffins: Increase grated lemon peel to 2 tablespoons and add 1 tablespoon poppy seeds.

Raspberry Muffins: Add 1 1/4 cups fresh, gently washed raspberries and 1 teaspoon ground cinnamon.

Breakfast Sausage
by Carol Fenster, Ph.D. – *Special Diet Celebrations*, 1999
C, D, E, G, N, S

1 pound ground beef	1/2 teaspoon black pepper
1 teaspoon rubbed sage	1/2 teaspoon fennel seed
1/2 teaspoon salt	1/4 teaspoon ground nutmeg
1/2 teaspoon dried thyme	1/8 teaspoon ground cloves
1/2 teaspoon ground cumin	1/8 teaspoon cayenne pepper
1/2 teaspoon dried savory	

Blend all ingredients together in large bowl using your hands or a large spatula. Form into patties or links and fry on medium heat until browned. Or, simply brown mixture in skillet for crumbled sausage. Serves 12.

Calories 110; Fat 8g, Protein 0g, Carb 1g, Chol 36mg, Sodium 125mg, Fiber 1g

Granola
by Carol Fenster, Ph.D. – *Special Diet Celebrations*, 1999
C, D, E, G (use rice flakes), N, S

2 cups oatmeal* or rolled rice flakes	2 teaspoons canola oil
1/2 teaspoon ground cinnamon	1/4 teaspoon salt
1/4 cup sesame seeds	1/4 cup honey
1/2 cup sunflower seeds	1/4 cup golden raisins
1/4 cup unsweetened coconut flakes	1/2 cup dried fruit of choice
1 teaspoon vanilla extract	

Shake all ingredients together, except dried fruit, in large plastic container with a tight fitting lid or in a large plastic bag.

Spread granola on non-stick baking sheet. Bake at 300° for 30-40 minutes, or until lightly browned. Stir every 10 minutes for even browning. Remove from oven; cool 15 minutes. Add dried fruit. Cool, then store in airtight container in dark, dry place. Makes about 4 cups. Serves 8.

Calories 210; Fat 9g, Protein 4g, Carb 31g, Chol 1mg, Sodium 128mg, Fiber 3g

*Oats are not approved for gluten-sensitive persons. Rolled rice flakes are available from Nancy's Natural Foods (see Vendors in Appendix).

Dinnertime!

Dinnertime is the magic hour or—depending on your household—the hectic hour. These recipes will make dinnertime quick, easy, and satisfying for everyone.*

Meatloaf Par Excellence
by T. M. Willingham
C, D, E (use flax), G, N, S (with rice milk) Check ketchup ingredients.

Meatloaf
1 pound ground beef
1 egg or 1/4 cup flax mix*
1/2 cup gluten-free bread
   crumbs (see page 216)
1/2 teaspoon dried sage
1 small onion, chopped fine
1 clove garlic, minced
*See page 231

1/3 cup soy or rice milk
1/2 teaspoon salt
1/4 teaspoon pepper

Topping
1 cup ketchup
1/3 cup brown sugar
1 tablespoon cider vinegar

Heat oven to 375°. Combine meatloaf ingredients. Shape into lightly greased loaf pan. Combine topping ingredients and spoon over meatloaf. Bake 60 minutes or until done. Serves 6.
Calories 360; Fat 22g; Protein 16g; Carb 27g; Chol 94; Sodium 870; Fiber 2g

Picadillo
by T.M. Willingham
C, D, E, G, N, S

1 pound ground beef
1 small onion, chopped fine
1 clove garlic, minced
1/2 teaspoon cumin
1/2 teaspoon oregano

1/4 teaspoon chili powder
2 baking potatoes, cubed
1 tablespoon olive oil
1 tomato, diced
12 olives, sliced thin

Sauté ground beef and onion. Add garlic and spices and cook until well done. Fry potatoes in olive oil until brown. Add to ground beef mixture, along with tomato and sliced olives. Simmer for 20 minutes. Serves 8. Serve with rice and beans.
Calories 230; Fat 18g; Protein 10g; Carb 7g; Chol 48mg; Sodium 170mg; Fiber 1g

*For more main dishes, see Carol Fenster's cookbooks (in Bibliography).

Rice and Black Beans, Cuban style
by T.M. Willingham
E, D, G, N, S

1 can (15 oz.) black beans
2 tablespoons olive oil
1 tablespoon cider vinegar
1 clove garlic, minced

1 1/2 teaspoons oregano
1 teaspoon marjoram
2 cups cooked white rice

Rinse and drain beans. Add olive oil, vinegar, garlic, oregano, and marjoram. Stir well. Microwave on high for two minutes. Stir again before serving. Serve over white rice. Serves 4.

Calories 550; Fat 9g; Protein 26g; Carb 95g; Chol 0mg; Sodium 8mg; Fiber 17g

Chicken à la Chris
by T.M. Willingham
D, E, G, N, S

6 boneless chicken breast
   halves or tenderloins
1 medium egg, beaten*
1/4 cup soy or rice milk
***See page 216

1 bag (4 oz.) Salad Eatos** corn
   croutons (crushed) or 1 cup
   gluten-free bread crumbs***
2 teaspoons fresh lemon juice

Heat oven to 375°. Lightly grease 9 x 9-inch baking pan. Mix beaten egg and milk together and submerge chicken pieces in it, then dredge in crumbs. Arrange in single layer in baking pan. Drizzle with lemon juice. Bake 30-40 minutes, or until chicken browns and juices run clear. Serves 6.

Calories 210; Fat 4g; Protein 31g; Carb 13g; Chol 95mg. Sodium 200mg; Fiber 1g

*For egg-free version, omit egg and dip chicken in soy or rice milk only
** Made by R.W. Garcia/Santa Cruz Foods. Available at grocery stores in a variety of seasoned flavors, including tomato, basil, and ranch. This is Chris' favorite recipe, hence the name.
***See page 216.

Taco Tatos
by T.M. Willingham
C, D, E, G, N, S

1 pound ground beef	1 teaspoon oregano
1 small onion, chopped fine	1/2 teaspoon marjoram
1 clove garlic, minced	1/4 teaspoon cumin
2 teaspoons chili powder	4 large baking potatoes, baked

Brown ground beef, onion, garlic, and spices over medium heat. While browning meat, microwave 4 large baking potatoes. (If you bake them in the oven, start at least an hour ahead of time.) Serve meat mixture over baked potatoes. Serves 4. Optional toppings (if safe for your diet): sour cream, salsa, grated cheese, etc.

Calories 450; Fat 30g; Protein 22g; Carb 23g; Chol 96mg; Sodium 230; Fiber 3g

Southwestern Style Rice and Beans
by T.M. Willingham
D, E, G, N, S

1 can (16 oz.) red kidney beans	1 package (1 lb.) frozen corn
1 cup cooked white rice	1/4 cup salsa

Prepare white rice as directed. Rinse and heat kidney beans. Prepare frozen corn as directed. Mix rice, kidney beans, and corn, add salsa and serve. (For a corn-free dish, replace corn with a mixture of chopped red or green peppers or tomatoes or use another can of beans.) Serves 4.

Calories 500; Fat 3g; Protein 29g; Carb 99g; Chol 0mg; Sodium 29mg; Fiber 19g

211

Pizza Crust & Pizza Sauce

by Carol Fenster, P h. D. – *From Special Diet Celebrations*, 1999
C (check tomato sauce), D, E, G, N, S

Pizza Crust

1 tablespoon dry yeast
1 1/4 cups Mix #1 or #2 (page 177)
2 teaspoons xanthan gum
1/2 teaspoon salt
1 teaspoon unflavored gelatin
1 teaspoon Italian seasoning

2/3 cup warm (110°) soy or rice milk
1 teaspoon sugar or honey
1 teaspoon olive oil
1 teaspoon cider vinegar
Extra rice flour for sprinkling

Pizza Sauce

1 can (8 oz.) tomato sauce
1/2 teaspoon dried oregano
1/2 teaspoon dried basil
1/2 teaspoon dried rosemary
1/2 teaspoon fennel seeds

1 garlic clove, minced
2 teaspoons sugar
1/2 teaspoon salt
Toppings of your choice

Sauce: Combine all ingredients in small saucepan and bring to boil over medium heat. Reduce heat to low and simmer for 15 minutes, while Pizza Crust is being assembled. Makes 1 cup.

Crust: Preheat oven to 425°. In medium mixer bowl using regular beaters (not dough hooks), blend the yeast, flour mix, xanthan gum, salt, gelatin powder, and Italian seasoning on low speed. Add warm liquid, sugar, oil, and vinegar.

Beat on high speed for 3 minutes. (If the mixer bounces around, add water, one tablespoon at a time, until dough does not resist beaters.) Dough should resemble soft bread dough.

Put mixture on 12-inch pizza pan or baking sheet that has been generously greased. Liberally sprinkle rice flour onto dough, then press dough into pan, continuing to sprinkle dough with flour to prevent sticking to your hands. Make edges thicker to hold the toppings.

Bake pizza crust 10 minutes. Remove from oven. Top with sauce and toppings. Bake another 20-25 minutes or until top is nicely browned. Serves 6 (1 slice per serving).

Calories, 153; Fat 1.5g, Protein 4g; Carb. 33g; Chol.1 mg; Sodium 635 mg; Fiber 3g

Chicken Fingers
by Carol Fenster, Ph.D. – from a forthcoming book
C, D, E, G, N, S

4 boneless, skinless chicken
  breast halves
1 egg, beaten*

1/2 cup soy or rice milk
Breading Mix (see below)
1/4 cup canola oil (for frying)

Slice each chicken breast diagonally into 1/2-inch wide strips. Whisk together egg and milk. Dip each strip into egg mixture, then into breading mix. Fry in oil until browned. Add salt and pepper to taste. Or, bake on non-stick sheet at 350° for 30 minutes or until nicely browned. Serves 4.

Calories 270; Fat 16g; Protein 28g; Carb 1g; Chol 110mg; Sodium 90mg; Fiber 1g

*Egg-Free Chicken Sticks: Omit egg and dip chicken in soy or rice milk only.

Breading Mix
by Carol Fenster, Ph.D. – from a forthcoming book
C, D, E, G, N, S

1 cup potato (not starch) flour
1 cup arrowroot
1 teaspoon dried thyme
1 teaspoon dried oregano
1 teaspoon onion powder
*Featherweight brand

1 teaspoon baking powder*
1 teaspoon salt
1/2 teaspoon cayenne pepper
1/4 teaspoon garlic powder
1/4 teaspoon sugar

Mix ingredients together and store in airtight container in dark, dry place. Use as breading mix for meats, seafood, or vegetables in frying and baking. Do not reuse mix after dipping. Use within 3 months. Makes 2 cups.

Calories per tablespoon: 35; Fat 0g; Protein 1g; Carb 8g; Chol 0mg; Sodium 80mg; Fiber 1g.

Side Dishes
Side dishes add important fiber, nutrients, and flavor to meals.*

Scalloped Potatoes
by Carol Fenster, Ph.D. – *Wheat-Free Recipes & Menus*, 1999
C, D, E, G, N

4 medium russet potatoes (peeled, sliced)	1 tablespoon canola oil
3/4 teaspoon onion salt	2 tablespoons potato starch or sweet rice flour
1/4 teaspoon white pepper	2 cups soy or rice milk
1 tablespoon onion flakes	1 tablespoon Parmesan cheese
1/8 teaspoon ground nutmeg	(cow, rice, or soy - optional)
1/2 teaspoon dried mustard	Paprika for garnish

Preheat oven to 350°. Toss potatoes with salt, pepper, and onion flakes in 1 1/2-quart casserole or baking dish. Shake remaining ingredients in screw top jar and pour over potatoes. Sprinkle with paprika. Bake 1 hour or until browned. Serves 4.
Calories 170; Fat 6g; Protein 6g; Carb 23; Chol 0mg; Sodium 343mg; Fiber 3g

Scalloped Potatoes With Ham: Add 1 cup cubed ham and reduce onion salt to 1/2 teaspoon. Serves 4.
Calories 230; Fat 10g; Protein 12g; Carb 25g; Sod 700mg; Chol 2mg; Fiber 2g

Sweet Potato Chips
by T. M. Willingham
C, D, E, G, N, S

3 sweet potatoes in 1/2-inch slices	1/4 teaspoon cinnamon
1/4 cup canola oil	1 teaspoon sugar

Fry slices in single layer in oil over medium heat. Turn often, they burn quickly. Cool on paper towels, sprinkle with cinnamon and sugar (and a dash of salt). Serve hot. Serves 8.
Calories 100; Fat 7g; Protein 1g; Carb 9g; Chol 0mg; Sodium 5mg; Fiber 1g

*For more side dishes, see Carol Fenster's three cookbooks (in Bibliography).

Cabbage Coleslaw
by Carol Fenster, Ph.D. – *Special Diet Celebrations*, 1999
C, D, E, G, N, S

1 small cabbage, in chunks	2 teaspoons ground mustard*
1 medium carrot, in chunks	1/3 cup canola oil
1 bunch green onions (chopped)	1/2 teaspoon celery seed
2 tablespoons cider vinegar	1/2 teaspoon salt
3 tablespoons fresh lemon juice	1/4 teaspoon white pepper
1 teaspoon honey	1/4 teaspoon paprika

*Grind mustard seeds in coffee grinder

In food processor, combine all ingredients—except paprika. Pulse on/off until desired texture is reached. Transfer to serving bowl to chill. Garnish with paprika. Serves 4.

Calories 250; Fat 19g, Protein, 4g; Carb. 20g, Chol. 0mg, Sodium 410 mg, Fiber 8g

Sumptuous Succotash
by T.M. Willingham
D, E, G, N, S (use rice milk)

1 box (10 oz.) frozen lima beans	1 tablespoon canola oil
1 box (10 oz.) frozen corn	1/4 teaspoon salt
1/4 cup soy or rice milk	1/8 teaspoon black pepper

Cook frozen corn and limas as directed on the package. Mix together with milk, butter, salt, and pepper. Serves 6.

Calories 125; Fat 3g; Protein 5g; Carb 22g; Chol 0mg; Sodium 116mg; Fiber 3g

Vegetable Casserole
by Carol Fenster, Ph.D. – from a forthcoming book
C (unless you use corn), D, E, G, N

1 package (10 oz.) frozen
  vegetables of choice
1 1/2 cups chicken broth or
  soy or rice milk
2 tablespoon canola oil
1/4 cup onion soup mix
  (page 231)

1 teaspoon dried basil
1/4 teaspoon salt
2 tablespoons sweet rice flour
3/4 cup seasoned breadcrumbs
  (see below for gluten-free version)
1/4 cup Parmesan cheese
  (cow, rice, soy—optional)

Preheat oven to 375°. Grease 8 x 8-inch pan. Arrange vegetables in pan. Set aside.

Combine broth (reserve 1/4 cup), oil, onion soup mix, basil, and salt in small pan over medium heat. In small bowl, stir together reserved broth and sweet rice flour until smooth. Gently whisk into hot broth, stirring until mixture thickens.

Pour over vegetables. Top with crumbs and Parmesan cheese (if using). Bake 20-25 minutes or until bubbly. Serves 4.

Calories 280; Fat 12g; Protein 13g; Carb 33g; Chol 6mg; Sodium 2200; Fiber 5g

Seasoned Bread Crumbs
by Carol Fenster, Ph.D. – *Special Diet Celebrations*, 1999
C, D, E, G, N, S (check bread)

4 cups gluten-free bread
  (cut in cubes) (Or use regular
  bread if not gluten-sensitive)

4 teaspoons Italian herb
  seasoning (or 1 teaspoon
  each basil, oregano, rosemary and onion powder)

Place bread crumbs in food processor and pulse on/off until crumbs are desired consistency. Toss with seasoning. Store in tightly covered container in freezer for up to two months. To toast breadcrumbs, gently brown in 300° oven until light golden color. Makes about 2 cups.

Calories 55; Fat 1g; Protein 2g; Carb 10g; Chol 0mg; Sodium 95mg; Fiber 1g

Desserts
Dazzle the doubtful with these fabulous mouthfuls!*

Applesauce Cake
by Carol Fenster, Ph.D. – *Special Diet Celebrations*, 1999
C, D, E (without eggs), G, N, S (if not using tofu)

1 cup Mix #1 or #2 (page 177)
1/2 teaspoon xanthan gum
1 teaspoon unflavored gelatin
1/2 teaspoon salt
1 1/2 teaspoons baking soda
1 1/2 teaspoons baking powder*
1 teaspoon ground cinnamon
1/2 teaspoon ground cloves
*Featherweight brand
**See page 231

1/4 teaspoon ground nutmeg
1/4 teaspoon ground allspice
1 cup currants or raisins
1/4 cup canola oil
2/3 cup brown sugar
2 large eggs, 1/2 cup soft silken
   tofu or 1/2 cup flax mix**
1/2 cup applesauce
1 tablespoon cider vinegar

Preheat oven to 350°. Generously grease 6-cup nonstick Bundt cake pan or 8 x 8-inch nonstick cake pan.

Sift dry ingredients together (flour through allspice). In large mixing bowl, cream oil, sugar, egg (or tofu or flax), applesauce, and vinegar until thoroughly blended and very smooth. Slowly add dry ingredients, mixing just until combined. Fold in currants or raisins (dusted with flour mix).

Transfer to prepared pan. Bake for 25-30 minutes. Cool in pan 5-10 minutes. Remove cake and cool on wire rack. Serves 8.
Calories 250 Fat 10g, Protein 5g, Carb 33g, Chol 45mg, Sod 550mg, Fiber 2g

Easy Peanut Butter Cookies
by Nigel Dobson-Keeffe
C, D, G, S (check nut butter)

1 cup peanut butter (or butter
   from almonds, cashews, or
   sunflower or sesame seeds)

1 cup sugar
1 egg
1 teaspoon vanilla

Mix well and drop by 8 spoonfuls on cookie sheets. Bake at 350° for 9 minutes. Cool thoroughly. Makes 8 cookies.
Calories 300; Fat 17g; Protein 9g; Carb 32g; Chol 23g; Sodium 160; Fiber 2g
*For more dessert recipes, see Carol Fenster's three cookbooks (in Bibliography).

Chocolate Chip Cookies
by Carol Fenster, Ph.D. – *Special Diet Solutions*, 1998
C, D, E, G, N (check chocolate chips and margarine for corn and dairy)

1 1/2 cups Mix #1 or #2 (page 177)
1 teaspoon xanthan gum
1/2 teaspoon baking soda
1/4 teaspoon salt
1/4 cup margarine or spread
(free of corn, dairy, and soy)
3/4 cup brown sugar, packed
*See page 231

1/3 cup granulated sugar
2 teaspoons vanilla extract
1 extra large egg or 1/4 cup
flax mix*
1 cup chocolate chips
(no corn or dairy)
1/4 cup chopped nuts
(optional)

Preheat oven to 350°. Mix together flour, xanthan gum, baking soda, and salt. Set aside. Generously grease non-stick cookie sheet or use parchment paper. Set aside.

In large bowl of mixer, beat margarine (room temperature) with sugars, vanilla, and egg (or flax mix), scraping sides of bowl frequently. Beat in flour mixture on low speed, mixing thoroughly. Stir in chocolate chips (and nuts, if using). Drop by tablespoonfuls on baking sheet.

Bake on center rack of oven for 10-12 minutes, or until lightly browned or tops start to crack. Cool for 2-3 minutes before removing from cookie sheet. Makes 24 cookies.

Calories 120; Fat 5g; Protein 1g; Carb 20g; Chol 8mg; Sodium 76mg; Fiber 1g

Chocolate Chip Bars: Press mixture into greased 8 x 8-inch nonstick pan. Bake at 350° for 25-30 minutes. Cool before cutting.

Double Chocolate Chip Cookies: Replace 1/3 cup flour mix with unsweetened cocoa (not Dutch or alkali). Bake as directed.

Raisin Cookies: Replace chocolate chips with 1 cup dark raisins. Bake as directed.

Craisin® Cookies: Replace chocolate chips with 1 cup Craisins® (dried sweetened cranberries).

"Oatmeal" Cookies
C, D, E, G (if using rice flakes), N, S
by Carol Fenster, Ph.D. - *Special Diet Celebrations*, 1999

1 1/4 cups Mix #1 or #2 (page 177)
1/4 cup potato (not starch) flour
1/2 cup brown sugar
1/2 teaspoon salt
1/2 teaspoon xanthan gum
1/2 teaspoon baking soda
1/2 teaspoon baking powder*
1 teaspoon ground cinnamon
1 egg or 1/4 cup flax mix (page 231)

1/2 cup applesauce
2 tablespoons molasses
1 teaspoon vanilla extract
1/2 cup rolled rice flakes**
3/4 cup raisins

*Featherweight brand
**Available from Nancy's Natural Foods. (See Appendix). Rolled oats may be used if gluten is safe for your diet.

Preheat oven to 325°. Coat nonstick cookie sheet with cooking spray (or line with parchment paper). Set aside.

Combine dry ingredients and set aside.

In food processor, combine egg (or flax mix), applesauce, molasses, and vanilla extract until well blended.

Add dry ingredients and rolled rice flakes. Pulse until thoroughly mixed. Gently stir in raisins. Dough will be stiff.

Drop by tablespoons (or use spring-action ice cream scoop for evenly shaped cookies) onto prepared cookie sheet. Flatten each cookie to 1/2-inch thickness with wet spatula.

Bake 20-25 minutes or until edges begin to brown. For a flavor twist, add 1/3 cup nut butter of your choice like almond, cashew, or soy (if safe for your diet). Makes 12 cookies.

Calories 180; Fat 8g; Protein 2g; Carb 28g; Chol 25mg; Sodium 240mg; Fiber 2g

Oatmeal Cookie Bars: Press mixture into greased 8 x 8-inch nonstick pan. Bake at 325° for 25-30 minutes or until edges begin to brown. Cool completely before cutting.

219

Basic Yellow Cake

By Carol Fenster, Ph.D. – *Special Diet Celebrations*, 1999
C, D, E (without eggs), G, N, S (without tofu)

1/3 cup canola oil
1 cup sugar
2 large eggs or 1/2 cup soft
  silken tofu or flax mix*
1 tablespoon grated lemon peel
1 1/2 cups Mix #1 or #2 (page 177)
1 teaspoon xanthan gum
*See page 231

1/2 teaspoon baking powder**
1/2 teaspoon baking soda
1/4 teaspoon salt
1/4 cup soy or rice milk
2 teaspoons cider vinegar
1 teaspoon vanilla extract
**Featherweight brand

Preheat oven to 325°. Generously grease two 8-inch round pans and line with parchment paper or waxed paper. Or, use two 5 x 3-inch small cake pans. Set aside.

With electric mixer and large mixer bowl, cream together oil, sugar, eggs (or tofu or flax), and grated lemon peel on medium speed until thoroughly blended.

In a medium bowl, whisk together flour mix, xanthan gum, baking powder, baking soda, and salt. In mixing cup, combine milk, vinegar, and vanilla extract.

On low speed, beat dry ingredients into oil mixture, alternating with milk—beginning and ending with dry ingredients. Mix just until combined. Spoon batter into prepared pan(s) and smooth tops.

Bake 8-inch cakes for about 30-35 minutes or small loaf pans for 30-40 minutes—or until tops are golden brown and tester inserted in center comes out clean. Let cakes cool in pans for 5 minutes, then remove from pan, remove paper, and cool on rack. Serves 12.

Calories 195, Fat 6g, Protein 2g, Carb 33g, Chol 35mg, Sodium 144mg, Fiber 1g

Yellow Cake Cupcakes: Bake 12 cupcakes for 20-25 minutes.

Pineapple Upside-Down Cake: Place 1/2 cup brown sugar and a layer of pineapple slices (drained) in pan. Top with batter. Bake as directed.

Basic Chocolate Cake
By Carol Fenster, Ph.D. – *Special Diet Celebrations*, 1999
C, D, E (without egg), G, N, S (without tofu or soy milk)

1 1/2 cups Mix #1 or #2 (page 177)	2 teaspoons vanilla extract
1/2 cup cocoa (not Dutch)	1/2 cup soy or rice milk
1 teaspoon xanthan gum	1/3 cup canola oil
1 1/4 teaspoons baking soda	1 large egg or 1/4 cup soft
3/4 teaspoon salt	silken tofu or flax mix*
1 cup brown sugar	3/4 cup warm (105°) water
	*See page 231

Preheat oven to 350°. Generously grease 9-inch round non-stick pan or 11 x 7-inch nonstick pan. Set aside.

Place all ingredients, except hot water or coffee, in large bowl and blend with electric mixer. Add hot water and mix until thoroughly blended. Pour into prepared pan and bake for 30-35 minutes or until toothpick placed in center of cake comes out clean. Serves 12.

Calories 210, Fat 9g, Protein 2g, Carb. 33g, Chol. 38mg, Sodium 300mg, Fiber 2g

Chocolate Cupcakes: Bake 12 cupcakes for 20-25 minutes.

Chocolate Layer Cake: Double recipe and bake in two 9-inch round nonstick pans for 35-40 minutes, or two 8-inch round nonstick pans for 25-30 minutes or until tester inserted in center comes out clean. For easier cake removal, spray pan(s) with cooking spray first, then line with waxed paper or parchment paper. Then spray again. Use cooking spray that is safe for your diet.

Chocolate Raspberry Cake: Reduce water to 2 tablespoons and add 1/2 cup thoroughly crushed raspberries.

221

Sugar Cookies
By Carol Fenster, Ph.D. – *Special Diet Celebrations*, 1999
C, D, E, G, N (check spread ingredients for corn or dairy)

1/4 cup margarine or spread	1/2 teaspoon xanthan gum
2 tablespoons honey	1/2 teaspoon salt
1/2 cup sugar	1 teaspoon baking powder*
1 teaspoon vanilla extract	1/2 teaspoon baking soda
2 teaspoons grated lemon peel	2 tablespoons water (if needed)
1 1/2 cups Mix #1 or #2 (page 177)	Additional rice flour for rolling
	*Featherweight brand

In food processor, combine margarine (room temperature, not melted), honey, sugar, vanilla, and lemon peel. Process for 1 minute. Add flour mix, xanthan gum, salt, baking powder, and baking soda, blending all ingredients until mixture forms large clumps. Scrape down sides of bowl with spatula and blend until mixture forms ball again. Add water only if necessary—1 tablespoon at a time. Refrigerate, covered, 3 to 4 hours.

Preheat oven to 325°. For cut out cookies: using one-half of the dough, roll to 1/4-inch thickness between sheets of waxed paper or plastic wrap which are sprinkled with rice flour. Keep remaining dough chilled until ready to use. Cut into desired shapes (about 2 inches in diameter) and transfer to baking sheet sprayed with cooking spray or lined with parchment paper or non-stick baking liners. Place about 2 inches apart.

For regular cookies, roll into 16 walnut-shaped balls and place on prepared sheet about 2 inches apart.

Bake 10-12 minutes, or until cookies are lightly browned. Cool 2 minutes on pan. Remove from cookie sheet and cool on wire rack. Makes 16.

Calories 90, Fat 3g, Protein .5g, Carb 15g, Chol 0mg, Sodium 71mg, Fiber .5g

Suggestions for Cut-Out Cookies: Christmas: angel, bell, candy cane, tree, reindeer, star; **Halloween**: cats, half-moon, leaf, owl, pumpkins, witches; **Southwestern:** cactus, howling wolf; **Thanksgiving**: pumpkins, turkey; **Spring/Easter:** bunny, butterfly, chick, tulip; **St. Patrick's Day:** shamrock; **Valentine's Day:** flower, heart

Tips For Successful "Cut-Out" Cookies
Using Sugar Cookie Recipe on Previous Page

1. To avoid sticking, use non-stick baking liners or parchment paper.
2. Insulated baking sheets assure even baking and won't buckle.
3. Metal cookie cutters work better than plastic cookie cutters.
4. If the chilled dough is too stiff, leave dough at room temperature for 15-20 minutes. Then knead with hands to make dough more pliable. If dough is too soft after rolling, chill or freeze until firm—then cut into desired shapes. Do not roll dough thinner than 1/4 inch.
5. If you're having trouble transferring the cookies to the baking sheet, try rolling the dough onto parchment paper or nonstick liners, cut desired shapes, remove scraps of dough (leaving cut-out cookies on paper) and transfer paper or liner (cookies and all) to baking sheet.

Snickernoodles: Use a tablespoon to shape dough into 16 walnut-size balls. Roll in mixture of 2 tablespoons sugar and 1 teaspoon cinnamon. Bake as directed.

Peanut Butter Cookies: Replace 1/4 cup margarine with 1/4 peanut butter (or other butter made from almond, cashews, soy—if safe for your diet—or sunflower seeds). Bake as directed.

Lemon Cookies: Add 2 tablespoons grated lemon peel to dough. Bake as directed.

Pecan Cookies: Add 1/4 cup finely chopped pecans (if safe for your diet) or sunflower seeds to dough. Bake as directed.

Coconut Cookies: Add 1/4 cup finely shredded coconut to dough. Bake as directed.

Spice Cookies: Add 1 teaspoon cinnamon and 1/2 teaspoon ginger to dough (or your preferred spices). Bake as directed.

223

Coconut Crusted Ice Cream Pie
by Carol Fenster, Ph.D. – *Special Diet Celebrations*, 1999
C, D (without ice cream), E, G, N (use pumpkin seeds), S

Crust
1 1/2 cups shredded coconut
1 tablespoon sweet rice flour
1/4 teaspoon salt
1 teaspoon vanilla extract
2 tablespoons canola oil

Pie Filling
1 pint ice cream or frozen sorbet

Toppings of Your Choice

Crust: Oil a 9-inch pie plate. Combine ingredients thoroughly and press onto bottom and up sides. Bake at 325° until lightly toasted, approximately 10-15 minutes. Watch carefully so crust doesn't burn. Freeze.

Filling: Spread softened ice cream or sorbet into crust. Freeze. Serve with your favorite toppings. Serves 10.

Calories (Crust only) 56; Fat 2g; Protein 1g; Carb 8g; Chol 0mg; Sodium 80mg; Fiber 0g

Cobbler Topping
by Carol Fenster, Ph.D. – *Special Diet Celebrations*, 1999
C, D, E, G, N, S

1 cup Mix #1 or #2 (page 177)
1 teaspoon xanthan gum
1/2 teaspoon baking soda
1/2 teaspoon baking powder*
1/4 teaspoon salt
1/3 cup soy or rice milk
*Featherweight brand

2 tablespoons canola oil
2 tablespoons honey
1 teaspoon vanilla extract
1 teaspoon grated lemon peel
Fruit Filling of Choice

In large bowl, combine flour, xanthan gum, baking soda, baking powder, and salt. In another bowl, whisk together milk, oil, honey, vanilla, and lemon peel. Add to dry ingredients, stirring just until dry ingredients are moistened. Drop by rounded tablespoons onto fruit filling.

Bake in middle of oven for 20-25 minutes or until filling is bubbly and crust is golden. Serve warm. Serves 6.

Calories (Topping): 35; Fat 4g; Protein 3g; Carb 20g; Chol 1mg; Sodium 290mg; Fiber 1g

Chocolate Brownies
C, D, E, G, N (omit walnuts), S

1 cup Mix #1 or #2 (page 177)
1/2 cup unsweetened cocoa
  (not Dutch)
1/2 teaspoon baking powder*
1/2 teaspoon salt
1/2 teaspoon xanthan gum
1/4 cup canola oil
*Featherweight brand

1/2 cup brown sugar, packed
1/2 cup granulated sugar
1 large egg**
2 teaspoons vanilla
1/4 cup hot water
1/2 cup chopped walnuts
  (optional)

Preheat oven to 350 degrees. Spray 8-inch square nonstick pan with cooking spray. Set aside.

Stir together the flours, cocoa, baking powder, salt, xanthan gum, instant coffee (if using), and egg replacer (if using egg-free recipe below). Set aside.

In large mixing bowl, beat the butter (or oil), sugars, egg (if using), and vanilla with electric mixer on medium speed until well combined. With mixer on low speed, add dry ingredients and hot water or coffee. Mix until just blended. Mixture will be somewhat thick. Stir in nuts, if using. Spread batter in prepared pan. Bake for 20 minutes. Cool brownies before cutting into 12 pieces. Serves 12.

** For egg-free brownies, omit egg and add 2 teaspoons Ener-G Egg Replacer powder. Increase hot water to 1/3 cup. Bake as directed.
Calories 180, Fat 6g; Protein 2g; Carb 33g; Chol 0mg; Sodium, 109mg; Fiber 1.5g

Nutty Rice Cereal Crust: (C, D, E, G, N, S) In food processor, blend 1 1/4 cups Pacific Grain® Nutty Rice Cereal, 3 tablespoons sugar, 1/8 teaspoon each ground cinnamon and nutmeg, and 1/3 cup canola oil until cereal is finely ground. Preheat oven to 325°. Press mixture into bottom and around sides of 9-inch pie plate. Serves 6.

Bake for 10 minutes. Cool before filling with pie filling.
Calories 190; Fat 13g; Protein 1g; Carb 19g; Chol 0mg; Sodium 30mg; Fiber 1g

Chocolate Pudding
by Carol Fenster, Ph.D. – *Special Diet Solutions*, 1998
C (use sweet rice flour), D, G, N, S (use rice milk)

1/2 cup sugar	1 3/4 cup soy or rice milk*
2 tablespoons cornstarch or	1 tablespoon canola oil
sweet rice flour	1 teaspoon vanilla
1/4 cup unsweetened cocoa	
1/8 teaspoon salt	

Combine sugar, cornstarch, cocoa, and salt in medium saucepan. Over medium heat, whisk in milk. Stir constantly until mixture thickens, about 5-8 minutes. Do not overcook.

Remove from heat and add oil and vanilla. Pour into individual custard cups or dessert bowls. Chill until firm. Serves 4 small servings (1/2 cup each).

*If using rice milk, dissolve 2 teaspoons unflavored gelatin in 1/4 cup of the milk for 10 minutes. Add with rest of milk. Cook as directed.

Calories 170, Fat 1 g, Protein 4g, Carb. 37g, Chol. 2mg, Sodium 220 mg, Fiber 1g

Flower Pot Treats: Layer chocolate pudding and crushed cookies (your choice) in clean, miniature flowerpots. Bury "worms" cut from pure fruit leather in pudding. Top with artificial flower to resemble flowerpots.

Chocolate Frozen Dessert: Prepare Chocolate Pudding as directed above. Chill. Process in electric ice cream maker. Serve as chocolate "ice cream".

NOTE: Electric ice cream makers work especially well for frozen desserts. I prefer the type with gel-filled canisters that you freeze before filling with prepared dessert. The canister sits on a base and rotates until the dessert is frozen. An alternative is to freeze individual servings in small paper cups.

Breads
Bread is an important part of *everyone's* diet.*

Corn Bread
by Carol Fenster, Ph.D. – *Special Diet Solutions*, 1998
D, E, G, N, S (with rice milk)

2/3 cup Mix #1 or #2 (page 177)
1/2 cup yellow cornmeal
2 tablespoons sugar
1/2 teaspoon xanthan gum
1 teaspoon baking powder*
1/2 teaspoon baking soda

1/2 teaspoon salt
1 large egg, lightly beaten*
2/3 cup soy or rice milk
2 teaspoons cider vinegar
2 tablespoons canola oil
*Featherweight brand

Generously grease 8-inch round or square nonstick pan. Set aside. Preheat oven to 350°.

In medium bowl, combine flour, cornmeal, sugar, xanthan gum, baking powder, baking soda, and salt (and egg replacer, if using). Make a well in center. Set aside.

In another bowl, beat egg (if using), milk, vinegar, and oil until well blended. Add to dry mixture, stirring just until moistened. Batter will be thick.

Bake for 20-25 minutes, or until top is firm and edges are lightly browned. (Or, bake the corn bread in 6-muffin tins for 20-25 minutes.) Serve warm. Serves 6.

Calories 350; Fat 9g; Protein 15g; Carb 20g; Chol 31mg; Sodium 260; Fiber 5g.

**Omit egg, add 1 tablespoon Ener-G egg replacer powder and increase soy or rice milk to 1 cup.

*For more bread recipes, see Carol Fenster's three cookbooks (in Bibliography).

Sandwich Bread

by Carol Fenster, Ph.D. – from a forthcoming book
C, D, E, G, N, S (with rice milk)

1 tablespoon dry yeast	1 teaspoon Ener-G egg
1 cup soy or rice milk	replacer
2 tablespoons sugar, divided	2 large eggs or 1/3 cup
2 1/2 cups Mix #1 or #2 (page 177)	flax mix (page 231)
2 teaspoons xanthan gum	3 tablespoons canola oil
1 teaspoon salt	1 teaspoon cider vinegar

Combine yeast, 2 teaspoons of the sugar, and warm (110°) water. Set aside to foam for 5 minutes.

In large bowl of heavy-duty, table-top mixer (300 watts or more) using beaters (not dough hooks), combine remaining ingredients, including remainder of sugar and yeast mixture.

Blend ingredients on low, then at medium speed for 2 minutes, scraping down sides of bowl with spatula as necessary. Place dough in greased 8 x 4-inch nonstick pan. Smooth top of dough with wet spatula. Cover and let rise in warm (75-80°) place until dough is level with top of pan (approximately 30-40 minutes).

BAKE at 375° for 50-55 minutes (do not underbake). Cover with foil after 10 minutes to prevent over-browning. Tap loaf with fingernail. A crisp, hard sound indicates a properly baked loaf. Turn loaf out on to wire rack and cool thoroughly before slicing with an electric knife or serrated knife. Makes a 1-pound loaf. Serves 10.

Calories 220; Fat 7g; Protein 6g; Carb 26g; Chol 36mg; Sodium 241mg; Fiber 2mg

Raisin Bread: Add 1 cup raisins, 1 tablespoon brown sugar, and 1 teaspoon cinnamon. Bake as directed.

Calories 270; Fat 7g; Protein 7g; Carb 38g; Chol 36mg; Sodium 244mg; Fiber 2.5mg

Note: Bread will be heavier and more dense without eggs.

Banana Bread

By Carol Fenster, Ph.D. – *Special Diet Solutions*, 1998
C, D, E (without eggs), G, N (use sunflower seeds), S

3 tablespoons canola oil
2/3 cup brown sugar, packed*
2 large eggs or 1/3 cup flax
mix (see page 231)
1 teaspoon vanilla extract
1 3/4 cup Mix #1 or #2
(#2 preferred)
1/2 teaspoon xanthan gum

1/2 teaspoon salt
2 teaspoons baking powder*
1 1/4 teaspoons cinnamon
1 1/2 cups mashed ripe bananas
1/2 cup chopped pecans or
sunflower seeds (optional)
1/2 cup raisins
*Featherweight brand

Preheat oven to 350°. Grease 9 x 5-inch nonstick pan. For smaller loaves, use two small loaf pans 5 x 3-inches each.

Cream oil, sugar, eggs (or flax), and vanilla together. Add flour, xanthan gum, salt, baking powder, and cinnamon to egg mixture, alternating with bananas. Stir in nuts (or seeds) and raisins. Batter will be somewhat soft. Transfer to pan(s).

Bake 9 x 5-inch loaf for 1 hour; 5 x 3-inch pans for 45 minutes. Serves 10.

Calories 285; Fat 9g; Protein 3g; Carb 50g; Chol 45mg; Sodium 245mg; Fiber 2g

Dressings, Condiments, and Miscellaneous
Spice up your diet with these allergen-free recipes.*

Creamy Italian Dressing
adapted from a recipe by Melissa Taylor - FAST
C, D, E, G, N, S

1/2 cup canola oil
1/2 cup Mock Mayonnaise (below)
1/3 cup water
2 tablespoons red wine vinegar
1 teaspoon each sugar and salt
1 teaspoon lemon juice

1/4 teaspoon xanthan gum
1/4 teaspoon onion powder
1/4 teaspoon dried parsley
1/4 teaspoon dried oregano
1/8 teaspoon cayenne pepper
1/8 teaspoon black pepper

Blend ingredients in blender. Chill. Makes 1 1/2 cups.

Mock Mayonnaise
by Melissa Taylor - FAST
C, D, E, G, N, S

1 cup water
1 cup canola oil
1 tablespoon lemon juice
1 tablespoon cider vinegar
1 tablespoon sugar
2 teaspoons arrowroot powder

1 teaspoon xanthan gum
1/2 teaspoon salt
1/4 teaspoon dry mustard*
1/8 teaspoon paprika
1/8 teaspoon cayenne
1/8 teaspoon onion salt

*Grind your own in coffee grinder for gluten-free version
Blend ingredients in blender. Refrigerate. Makes 2 cups.

Ranch Dressing
C, D, E, G, N, S (with rice milk)

1/2 cup Mock Mayonnaise (above)
1/2 cup soy or rice milk
1/4 teaspoon onion salt
1/8 teaspoon garlic salt

1/4 teaspoon each black
pepper, dried marjoram,
celery salt, dried savory,
and dried parsley

Whisk ingredients together. Refrigerate. Makes 1 cup.

All recipes on page: *Calories 55, Fat 5g; Protein 1g; Carb 1g; Chol 5mg; Sod 56mg, Fiber 0g*
* Unless otherwise noted, these recipes are from Carol Fenster's cookbooks (see Bibliography).

Flax (Flaxseed) Mix
C, D, E, G, N, S

3 teaspoons flaxmeal (if using flax-seeds, grind to powder with coffee grinder)   **1 cup boiling water**

Whisk flax into boiling water, remove from heat, and let stand for 5 minutes. Use as substitute for eggs—1/4 cup flax mix equals 1 large egg. (Baked items are heavier and denser.)
Calories 12, Fat 1g, Prot <1g, Carb 0g, Chol 0mg, Sod 3mg, Fiber 1g.

Onion Soup Mix
C, D, E, G, N, S (check bouillon)

1/2 cup dried minced onions
1 teaspoon onion salt
1/4 teaspoon garlic powder
1/4 teaspoon sugar

1 tablespoon sweet rice flour
1/2 teaspoon bouillon granules*
1/4 teaspoon apple pectin powder
*Ener-G brand is gluten-free

Combine ingredients in screw-top jar. Store in dark, dry place. Use in same proportions as commercial onion soup mix. Double or triple recipe, if needed.
Calories per tablespoon 20; Fat 0g; Protein 1g; Carb 5g; Chol 0mg; Sodium 203mg; Fiber 48g

White Sauce
C, D, E, G, N, S (with rice milk)

1 3/4 cups soy or rice milk
1/4 teaspoon onion powder
1 bay leaf
1/4 teaspoon salt
1/2 teaspoon dried thyme

1/4 teaspoon white pepper
1 tablespoon oil
2 tablespoons sweet rice flour
(dissolved in 3 tablespoons water)
Dash of ground nutmeg

In small saucepan over low-medium heat, bring milk, onion powder, bay leaf, salt, thyme, white pepper, and oil to simmer. Remove from heat and let stand for 10 minutes to blend flavors. Strain and discard solids. Stir in sweet rice flour mixture and continue whisking until thickened. Remove from heat. Add nutmeg. Makes 1 3/4 cups. Serves 6. (1/4 cup each)
Calories 55; Fat 4g; Protein. 2g; Carb. 4g; Chol. 6g; Sodium 109 mg; Fiber 0g

Gluten-Free Play Dough
C (use potato starch), D, E, G, N, S

1/2 cup brown rice flour
1/2 cup cornstarch or potato starch
1/2 cup salt
2 teaspoons cream of tartar

1 cup water
1 teaspoon canola oil
Food coloring (optional, or use natural colors available at health food stores)

Sift dry ingredients together, blend with water and oil, and stir on low heat for 3 minutes or a ball forms. Store in airtight can.

Additional Tips

1. Powder from ground vanilla beans may be used instead of vanilla extract. Some non-alcohol brands *may* contain corn.
2. Nutritional yeast may be used in place of Parmesan cheese. Soyco makes a lactose-free, soy-based Parmesan cheese, but the rice version has casein.
3. Agave nectar looks like honey. Buy it in health food stores.
4. Margarine or spreads that are free of both dairy and soy are hard to find. Read labels very carefully on these products.
5. Safflower or sunflower oil may be used in place of canola oil in sweet dishes. Olive oil may be used in savory dishes.
6. McCormick spices are usually gluten-free unless the offending ingredient is specifically listed on label.
7. Baking without eggs results in a heavier, more dense texture. When possible, use Mix #2 (bean flour) in egg-free baking.
8. Rice and soy milks (beverages) can differ in thickness or viscosity. Sometimes you'll need more… sometimes less. Some experimentation may be required!
9. If xanthan gum is not appropriate for your diet (it is grown on corn, yet used by the corn-sensitive), use half again as much guar gum instead.
10. If you can't find appropriate chocolate chips, chop up Chocolove brand pure chocolate, which is simply ground up cocoa beans.
11. Remember…read the labels on EVERY ingredient!

Chapter XII
Wheat-Free, Milk-Free, Peanut-Free, Egg-Free, Corn-Free, Soy-Free...Stress Free
The Last Word

When we first discovered Chris had a food sensitivity, we really didn't dwell on it too much. We learned what we could, from the limited amount of information available at the time, and then continued to educate ourselves on food sensitivities as we went along. Most of the time, though, we never even thought about it—at least not as an "illness," unless perhaps he was invited to a party, or a relative brought a forbidden food, or he looked longingly at a friend's birthday cake.

And when that happened, we adapted. We found cookbooks that featured wheat-free recipes; we learned to be spontaneous within our limits, to not worry about every little accidental ingestion. And, something else happened, too.

When we took wheat off the table for Chris and began looking at other types of foods, a whole new world opened up for us, a world outside speed and convenience—our culinary horizons opened up to the world of real, wholesome foods. We rediscovered fruits and vegetables, discovered new grains and flours for the first time, and discovered anew the joy of cooking thoughtfully and with an eye to health and well being.

Far from being the curse so many thought Chris' wheat sensitivity would be, it rained blessings down upon us we would never have imagined. Providing him with the foods he could eat in a way he enjoyed and watching him thrive and grow, symptom-free and happy, gave me the same sense of well-being and accomplishment that nursing him and his sisters when they were babies had given me. *I* was making him feel good and grow big and strong. It was a wonderful feeling.

233

And he was teaching me something at the same time. He was teaching me about adaptability and resourcefulness. His good-natured acceptance of his life and the conditions set upon him are inspirational. Because of Chris, we view life with a perspective we would never have had otherwise.

And he definitely raised my health-intelligence quotient. I never thought about food too much before we discovered Chris' condition. Our family simply ate the foods we enjoyed without giving the source of our health and well-being much thought. After we learned about food sensitivities, we began learning about food itself, its beauties and complexities, its most essential qualities, and its least essential ones.

Many of the other families I spoke with have experienced similar epiphanies. A food sensitivity, they're learning, is not the end of the world. It is the beginning of a new world, a world of health-conscious food choices that can restore us to an intimate connection with the things of the earth that bring us life.

If there is a silver lining to living with a food sensitivity, it is that it forces us to examine our lives, from its most basic and fundamental aspects to its most sublime. We can view food sensitivities as an inconvenience... or as paving the way to our children's healthy birthrights; their birthrights of good, clean foods that make them feel happy, healthy and safe, and that bring us a measure of comfort in being able to provide them that good life and to teach them how to sustain it.

What more can any of us ask, and what more can we give?

Appendix

Bibliography and Suggested Reading

Allergy, Asthma and Immunology Society of Ontario, Peanut Allergy–What You Need To Know, Downsview, Ontario M3N 1M1, March 2000

Allergy Awareness Association, Allergies at School: A Teacher's Guide, Inform New Zealand Ltd, Dec. 1999

American Academy of Allergy, Asthma,& Immunology, "Thioredoxin and Milk Allergy," Journal of Allergy and Clinical Immunology, 1999

American Academy of Pediatrics Red Book, 2000. Report of the Committee on Infectious Diseases

Anaphylaxis Campaign, Guidance for Caterers, Farnborough, Hampshire

Anderson, John A., M.D. "Milk, Eggs and Peanuts: Food Allergies in Children, "American Family Physician, Vol. 56, No. 5, Oct 1, 1997

Ascher, Henry, M.D., "Quality and Quantity of Grains in the European Diet," 9th International Celiac Symposium, Baltimore, MD, Aug 2000

Balch, James F., M.D. and Phyllis A. Balch, Prescription for Nutritional Healing, New York: Avery Publishing Group, 1997

Bovsun, Mara, "Vaccine May Prevent Peanut Allergy, " New York City, Washington, March 29 (UPI), MedServ Medical news, June 27, 1999

Buchanan, Robert, M.D., "How Research Using Plant Biotechnology Is Removing Allergens from Existing Foods," Senate Committee on Agriculture, Nutrition, &Forestry, Univ. of California, Berkeley, October 1999

Burks, Wesley, M.D. and John M. James, M.D., Mechanisms of Food Allergy, University of Arkansas Medical Sciences, Little Rock, AR

Brehler, R., et al., "Latex-fruit Syndrome: Frequency of Cross-Reacting IgE Antibodies," European Journal of Allergy/Clinical Immunology, April 1997

Cacciari E., et al.; "Short stature and celiac disease: a relationship to consider even in patients with no gastrointestinal tract symptoms," Journal of Pediatrics, 1983 Nov: 708-711

Calgary Allergy Network. Cross-Contamination: What is Peanut/Nut Free, Calgary, Canada.
---. A Guide for Parents/Students with Anaphylaxis,
---. Managing Food Allergies in the Classroom/Preparing Food Safely
---. Teacher's Guide to Allergy and Anaphylaxis,

Council for Responsible Nutrition. A Guide to Using Vitamin Supplements, Distributed with Assistance of Nat'l Association of Chain Drug Stores, 1999

Cowan, Doug, Psy. D., MFCC "Attention Deficit Hyperactivity Disorder Eating Program," ADD/ADHD information site.
<http://www.newideas.net/adddiet.htm>

Coyle, Joseph T., M.D., "Psychotropic Drug Use in Very Young Children," American Medical Association, March 2000

Crook, William G., M.D., The Yeast Connection Handbook, Professional Books, Inc., 2000
 -The Yeast Connection Cookbook: A Guide to Good Nutrition and
   Better Health (with Marjorie Hurt Jones, R.N.), Professional Books, 1998

Cruts, Jeni, "Milk Allergy Print-out," Food Allergy Survivors Together, FAST, 1998. <http://www.angelfire.com/mi/FAST >

"Family Dinner and Diet Quality Among Older Children and Adolescents," Journal of the American Medical Association, Vol. 9 No. 3, March 2000

Fasano, Alessio, M.D., "Study Launched To Discover Incidence Of Rarely Diagnosed Gastrointestinal Disorder," Center for Celiac Research at the University of Maryland Medical Center, Spring, 1998
---. "New Peanut Allergy Development," National Jewish Medical &
   Research Center, 1400 Jackson, Denver, Colorado, 80206
---. "Tissue Transglutaminase: The Holy Grail for the diagnosis of
   celiac disease, at last?," Journal of Pediatrics, 1999, 134-135
---. "Where Have All The American Celiacs Gone? "Arch Dis Child.,
   1996: 412:20-4
---. "Researchers Find Increased Zonulin Levels Among Celiac
   Disease Patients," Lancet, April 2000

Fenster, Carol, Ph.D., Special Diet Solutions, healthy cooking without wheat, gluten, dairy, eggs, yeast, or refined sugar, CO: Savory Palate, 1998
---. Wheat-Free Recipes & Menus: Delicious Dining Without Wheat
   or Gluten, CO: 1999
---. Special Diet Celebrations: no wheat, gluten, dairy, or eggs, CO: 1999

Fine, Kenneth, M.D., "Diagnosis of Gluten Sensitivity in the 21st Century: Time for A Change," Director of FinerHealth and Nutrition, and the Intestinal Health Institute Dallas, Texas <www.finerhealth.com>, EnteroLab www.enterolab.com

Garriott, Linda, M.S., R.D., C.D.E., "Corn", Texas Dept. of Health and Michelle E. Morat, Texas A&M University, February 2000

Gislason, Stephen, M.D., "Broad Overview of Celiac Disease," from Nutrition Therapy, Nutramed. <http://www.nutramed.com>

Groenewald, M.D., "Milk Allergy & Intolerance Information Sheet," Allergy Society of South Africa (ALLSA), Cape Town, RSA, 1999

Hasler, Clare, Ph.D., Soy and Human Health Web page

Hoffenberg, Edward, M.D., et al, "A Trial of Oats in Newly Diagnosed Celiac Disease," to be published Journal of Pediatrics, Children's Hospital, University of Colorado School of Medicine, Denver, 1999

Hoggan, Ronald, "Application of the Exorphin Hypothesis to Attention Deficit Hyperactivity Disorder: A Theoretical Framework," Dis. University Of Calgary, April 1998
---. "How Often is Short Stature Predictive of Celiac Disease?"

Hourihane, Jonathan O'B., M.D. et al., "An Evaluation of the Sensitivity of Subjects with Peanut Allergy to Very Low Doses of Peanut Protein: A Randomized, Double-Blind, Placebo-Controlled Food Challenge Study," Journal of Allergy and Clinical Immunology. November 1997

Internet Symposium on Food Allergens 1(4): 147-60 (1999) Allergen Data Collection: Rice (Oryza sativa). <http://www.food-allergens.de >

James, John M., M.D., Medical Advisory Board of Food Allergy Network, and Vice Chairman of the Adverse Reactions to Foods Committee for the American Academy of Allergy, Asthma, and Immunology, Fort Collins, CO

Janek J., and J.E. Simon (eds.) New Crops, Wiley, NY, 1993

Janatuinena, E.K., et al, "Oats Produce No Adverse Immunologic Effects in Patients With Celiac Disease, " Gut 2000; 46:327-331. March 10, 2000

Johns Hopkins Children's Center, "Researchers Close in on Source of Peanut Allergy, " Johns Hopkins Children's Center, November 22, 1996

Jones, Marjorie Hurt, R.N., Super Foods: Amaranth, Quinoa, Kamut, Buckwheat, Spelt, Teff, Coeur d'Alene, ID: MAST Enterprises, 1998

Kasarda, Donald D., Ph.D., "Celiac Disease," North American Society for Pediatric Gastroenterology and Nutrition, Toronto, ON, 1997

Korn, Danna, Kids with Celiac Disease: A Family Guide to Raising Happy, Healthy Gluten-Free Kids, Bethesda, MD: Woodbine, 2001

Lewis, Lisa S., Ph.D., "An Experimental Intervention For Autism: Understanding and Implementing a Gluten & Casein Free Diet,"© 1994, 1997. <http://members.aol.com/lisas156/gfpak.htm>
---. Special Diets for Special Kids, Future Horizons, 1998

Motala, Cassim, M. D., ALLSA -Food Allergy-Handbook, Allergy Society of South Africa, 1999. <http://allergysa.org/>

Nakase, M., et al., "Cereal Allergens: Rice-Seed allergens with Structural Similarity to Wheat and Barley Allergies," Allergy 53 (46 Suppl): 1998

National Institute of Allergy and Infectious Diseases, The National Institute of Allergy and Infectious Diseases of The National Institutes of Health. "Fact Sheet: Food Allergy and Intolerances, " April 1993. Revised January 1999

National Health and Medical Research Council, "Nhmrc Pamphlet On: Cows' Milk Intolerance In Children, Commonwealth of Australia, Sept 1996

Nelson, Roxanne, R.N., "How to Live with An Allergy to Soy", http://www. Ehow.com/eHow/eHow/0,1053,3966,FF.html

Ogawa, T., et al., "Investigation of the IgE-binding Proteins in Soybeans by Immunoblotting with the Sera of the Soybean-sensitive Patients with Atopic Dermatitis," Journal of Nutritional Science and Vitaminology, 1991

Oregon State University Extension Service, Cereals Specialist Russ Karow, "A Wheat Quality Primer", April 1998

Pruessner, Harold T., M.D, "Detecting Celiac Disease in Your Patients," American Family Physician, American Academy of Family Physicians, 1998

Quillan, Patrick, Ph.D., R.D., C.N.S, "Laws of Nutrition."

Scalise, Kathleen, "New Solution For Food Allergies Effective With Milk, Wheat Products, Maybe Other Foods, UC Researchers Discover, " News Release, 10/19/97, Regents of the University of California

Semrad, Carol E., M.D., "Celiac Disease and Gluten Sensitivity," Division of Digestive and Liver Diseases, Columbia University, 1995

Seroussi, Karyn and Bernard Rimland, Ph. D, Unraveling the Mystery of Autism and Pervasive Developmental Disorder: A Mother's Story of Research and Recovery, Simon and Schuster, February 2000

Sicherer, Scott H., M.D., "Manifestations of Food Allergy: Evaluation and Management," American Academy of Family Physicians, January 15, 1999

Snyder, O.P. and D. M. Poland, "Adverse Reactions to Food, Food Allergy and Sensitivity: A Retail Food Hazard Problem," Hospitality Institute of Technology and Management, St. Paul, MN, June 1997

Squires, Sally, "Increasing Incidence Of Peanut Allergy Puts Focus On Food-Reaction Hazards, Outwitting Allergens: Tips For Eating Safely," Washington Post, Oct. 23, 1996

Steinman, H.A., M.D., "Hidden Allergens in Foods," Journal of Allergy and Clinical Immunology 1996; 98(2): 241-250

Taylor, Steve L, Ph.D., "Prospects for the Future: Emerging Problems—Food Allergens," Conference on International Food Trade, October 1999

U.S. Food and Drug Administration, Center for Food Safety and Applied Nutrition, A Food Labeling Guide, September, 1994 (Ed. Rev., June, 1999)

Ventura, Alessandro, M.D., Celiac Disease and Autoimmunity: Which Comes First?", 9th Int'l Celiac Symposium, Baltimore, MD Aug 2000

Weisnagel, John, M.D., "Peanut Allergy: Where do we stand?, " October 1999, <http://www.allerg.qc.ca/peanutallergy.htm#prev>

Whelan, Ann, "Is Vinegar Safe for Celiacs?" Gluten-Free Living Sept/Oct. 1999
---. "More Thoughts on Vinegar," Gluten-Free Living, March/April 2000

Winter, Ruth, Consumer's Dictionary for Additives, Three Rivers, 1999

Wood, Rebecca, The Splendid Grain, William Morrow & Company, 1999

Corn-Sensitivity Fact Sheet
Food Allergy Field Guide (Savory Palate, 2000)
by Theresa Willingham

Corn sensitivity can result in skin rashes and asthma-like symptoms; the body's response to proteins it is unable to digest. In addition to avoiding obvious corn products like corn chips and tortillas, corn appears as a hidden allergen in countless foods that rely on corn-starch, corn meal, and corn syrup as thickeners and sweeteners. Ingredients like dextrose can be made from corn, as can maltodextrin, caramel, and malt syrup. Dextrose of an unknown source can be used in everything from French fries to fish sticks to caramel flavoring.

Corn can also be found in the adhesive in envelopes, stamps and stickers, in plastic wrap, paper cups and paper plates, although the latter are usually coated with corn oil, which usually causes no problems. Corn is also used to process aspirin, ointments, vitamins, and many toiletry items.

The corn-sensitive must also be alert for malt-type ingredients, any of which can be made from corn. Invert sugar, used in some candy and baked goods, is treated corn sugar. MSG is a famous corn derivative, known for producing unforgiving headaches in sensitive individuals. Any of the vague "vegetable" ingredients—vegetable protein, vegetable shortening, hydrolyzed vegetable protein and so forth—may contain corn.

⊘ AVOID	☑ OK
Dextrose.	Know exact source of dextrose.
Dextrin and maltodextrin .	Potato starch or other thickener.
Caramel flavoring .	Ask manufacturer for sources.
Corn syrup.	100% pure maple syrup, cane syrup, or beet sugars. Ask manufacturers for specifics.
Fructose is usually made of high fructose corn syrup.	Sucrose or sweeteners like maple or beet.
Invert syrup sugar is enzymatically treated bulk corn sugars.	Cane sugar, maple syrups, agave nectar.

⊘ AVOID	☑ OK
Cornstarch is added to most powdered sugars and baking powders to prevent clumping.	Corn-free powdered sugar from Miss Roben's. Corn-free baking powder by Featherweight.
Food starch, modified food starch, vegetable gum or starch.	Know food starch source.
Malt, malt syrup or malt extract.	Ask manufacturer for source
Mono- and diglycerides .	Ask manufacturer for source.
Monosodium glutamate .	Avoid MSG products.
Glucona delta lactone .	Avoid.
Marshmallows can contain corn	Ask manufacturer.
Vanilla extract typically contains corn syrup.	Ground vanilla bean powder
Xanthan gum	Guar gum, some intestinal distress for other reasons.
May **contain corn:**	**To maximize safety:**
Emollient creams.	Ask manufacturer for safe brand
Toothpastes.	Use non-allergenic toothpastes
Cosmetics.	Ask manufacturer for safe brand
Adhesives on envelopes, stamps.	Use self-stick
Aspirin.	Use alternative pain relievers
Laxatives.	Use natural laxatives or check with health food store.
Common brand name vitamins.	Use allergen free vitamins.
Bath powders.	Use all-talc powders, check with manufacturer to ensure safety.

For more information about Corn-Sensitivity:

American Academy of Asthma, Allergy & Immunology 611 E. Wells Street Milwaukee, WI 53202-3889 414.272.6071	American College of Allergy, Asthma, and Immunology 85 West Algonquin Road Arlington Heights, IL 60005
American Allergy Association P.O. Box 7273 Menlo Park, CA 94026 415.322.1663	Food Allergy Network 10400 Eaton Place, Suite 107 Fairfax, VA 22030-2208 800.929.4040; 703.691.2713 - fax www.foodallergy.org www.fankids.org (for kids)

Note: Be sure to check with your health professional about corn-free diets.

241

Dairy-Sensitivity Fact Sheet
Food Allergy Field Guide (Savory Palate, 2000)
by Theresa Willingham

According to the National Institutes for Health, as many as 30 to 50 million Americans are lactose intolerant, unable to digest the sugars in milk. Figures are higher for those of African or Asian descent, ranging from 75% of African Americans to 90% of Asian Americans. Cow milk allergy, an allergy to milk protein rather than sugar, can also cause problems. Milk sensitivities can cause breathing problems, hives and rashes, abdominal pain, diarrhea, and possibly serious weight loss.

⦸ AVOID	☑ OK
Milk solids ("curds"), whey.	Almond, oat, rice, and soy milk
Casein (sodium caseinate).	Avoid all caseinates
Lactose (sodium lactylate, frequently lactalbumin and other names that begin with lact)	Non-dairy beverages made without lactose..
"Natural" ingredients.	Know exact ingredient source.
Hydrolyzed vegetable protein.	Know exact source of protein.
"Non-dairy", e.g., Cool Whip	Read label for "non-dairy".
Kosher pareve desserts.	See below.
Canned tunafish.	Low sodium in spring water (StarKist), and Trader Joe tuna
Some chocolate candy.	Kosher pareve chocolates*.
Baked goods.	Unless certified safe through a known source, or homemade.
Processed or luncheon meats.	Check with manufacturer or buy non-processed meats only.
Ice cream; other dairy products.	Vegan alternatives.
Protein hydrolysates.	Ask manufacturer for source.

*Under most circumstances, Jewish dietary symbols on food packages are a reliable indicator of food content. If product is dairy, it will frequently have a D or the word Dairy next to the kashrut (the K in the circle or a K in a star) symbol). If it is pareve (made without milk, meat, or their derivatives) the word Pareve (or Parev) may appear near the symbol. However, the Food Allergy Network reminds us that the Pareve label may not ALWAYS be reliable. Milchig, another dietary law term, also means made of or derived from milk or dairy products.

Additional words which may denote dairy are: butterfat, butter oil, buttermilk, curds, custard, ghee, half-&-half, hydrolysates buttermilk, caseinates (ammonium, calcium, magnesium, potassium sodium), cheese, cream, cottage cheese, lactate solids, lactalbumin, lactalbumin phosphate, lactoglobulin, lactose, lactulose, milk solids, goat or sheep's milk, rennet casein, sour cream, whey, and yogurt.

Items which *may* include dairy are artificial butter flavor, artificial or natural flavors, bavarian cream, caramel, coconut cream, chocolate, non-dairy creamer, mayonnaise, margarine, nougat, pudding, sherbet, sorbet, and Simplesse©.

This above lists are constructed to avoid *both* sugar (lactose intolerance) and protein (e.g., cow milk allergy) in dairy products. However, experts remind us that lactose intolerant persons may tolerate small amounts of dairy such as cheese (which has smaller amounts of lactose than milk). Check with your physician.

For more information about Dairy sensitivities:

American Academy of Asthma, Allergy & Immunology 611 E. Wells Street Milwaukee, WI 53202-3889 414.272.6071	American Allergy Association P.O. Box 7273 Menlo Park, CA 94026 415.322.1663
American Dietetic Association 216 W. Jackson Boulevard Chicago, IL 60606-6995 800.745.0775 ext. 5000 http://www.eatright.org	American College of Allergy, Asthma, and Immunology 85 West Algonquin Road Arlington Heights, IL 60005
Bullseye Information Services 200 Linden Street, Dept. J Wellesley, MA 02181 508.647.0938	Food Allergy Network 10400 Eaton Place, Suite 107 Fairfax, VA 22030 800.929.4040; 703.691.3179 www.foodallergy.org www.fankids.org (for kids)
La Leche League International 1400 N. Meacham Road P.O. Box 4079 Schaumburg, IL 60168-4079 800.LALECHE	National Digestive Diseases Information Clearinghouse 2 Information Way Bethesda, MD 20892-3570 301.654.3810

Note: Be sure to check with your health professional about dairy-free diets.

243

Egg-Sensitivity Fact Sheet
Food Allergy Field Guide (Savory Palate, 2000)
by Theresa Willingham

Eggs are one of the most highly allergenic of foods, and even small amounts can cause reactions as severe as an anaphylactic reaction. Reactions can occur the very first time that a sensitive individual is exposed to the allergen. The culprit in egg sensitivity, as it is with many food sensitivities, is an inability to digest certain proteins. Symptoms of egg sensitivity can include allergic rhinitis, asthma, dermatitis, diarrhea and other gastrointestinal problems, hives, nausea, vomiting, itching of the mouth and tongue, wheezing and, at its most extreme, anaphylaxis.

Eggs are used frequently as binders, emulsifiers, and coagulants in foods, medicines, and toiletries. They appear in baked goods (often giving pretzels and cookies a shiny appearance), in sauces, candies, processed meats, dairy products of all kinds, pastas, sodas, and cereals. They're also in lotions, shampoos, ointments, and vaccines and other pharmaceuticals.

Here is a short list of what the egg-sensitive must avoid, but *due to the prevalence of eggs in so many items and the high danger of contamination in preparation facilities, the egg-sensitive should be especially careful when dining out. Restaurants are urged to be especially understanding of egg-sensitive diners' requests.*

⊘ AVOID	☑ OK
Albumin, ovalbumin, globulin, livetin, ovomucin, ovomucoid, silici albuminate, vitellin, ovovitellin.	*If unsure of any item, call manufacturer.*
Powdered egg, dried egg yolk, egg white.	*Pureed flaxseeds, pureed fruit, tofu, commercial egg replacer.*
Egg noodles.	*100% non-egg pasta.*
Milk puddings and custards.	*Egg-free custards and puddings.*
Pre- made pastries and breads.	*Make your own egg-free kind.*
Mayonnaise.	*Make your own egg-free kind.*
Lecithin	*Know exact source of lecithin.*

Other products which may contain eggs are: eggnog, globulin, livetin, lysozyme (used in Europe), mayonnaise, meringue, ovalbumin, ovomucin, ovomucoid, ovovitellin, Simplesse©, and vitellin. Any baked item with a shiny exterior may indicate the presence of eggs.

For more information about Egg Sensitivity:

American Academy of Allergy, Asthma, & Immunology 611 E. Wells Street Milwaukee, WI 53202-3889 414.272.6071	American College of Allergy, Asthma, and Immunology 85 West Algonquin Road Arlington Heights, IL 60005
American Allergy Association P.O. Box 7273 Menlo Park, CA 94026 415.322.1663	Food Allergy Network 10400 Eaton Place, Suite 107 Fairfax, VA 22030 800.929.4040; 703.691.3179 www.foodallergy.org www.fankids.org (for kids)
American Dietetic Association 216 W. Jackson Boulevard Chicago, IL 60606-6995 800.745.0775 ext. 5000 http://www.eatright.org	

Note: Be sure to check with your health professional about egg-free diets.

245

Peanut Sensitivity Fact Sheet
Food Allergy Field Guide (Savory Palate, 2000)
by Theresa Willingham

Sensitivity to peanuts typically manifests itself in a true allergic reaction, sometimes a serious one that can include anaphylactic episodes and death. Currently, it is believed that peanut allergy accounts for almost 30% of all food sensitivities, occurring most often in children under the age of 15 (who account for 93% of peanut allergy cases). It's also believed that peanut allergy accounts for the majority of food related anaphylaxis deaths in the U.S.

In the case of peanut sensitivity, a certain amount of hyper-vigilance is in order. Peanut residues on a counter top can cause asthma in certain individuals. Even the odor of peanuts has been known to cause allergic reactions in highly sensitive individuals. Peanuts are used in myriad ways, and are disguised under countless nom de plumes. Peanut butter can be used to thicken foods like chili, or to seal egg rolls. Peanuts can be altered and sold as other types of nuts. It's easy to contaminate baked goods or ice cream with peanuts.

Here is a short list of what the peanut-allergic must avoid, but *due to the prevalence of peanuts in so many items and the high danger of contamination in preparation facilities, the peanut sensitive should be especially careful when dining out. Restaurants should be especially understanding of peanut-sensitive diners' requests.*

⊘ AVOID	☑ OK
Mixed nuts.	*Use only nut sources you're sure of, and do not try to pick "safe" nuts from mixed nuts container.*
Peanut Butter.	*Soy, sunflower, or sesame (tahini) butter, from clean processing facilities.*
Legumes.	*If you know these are safe.*

246

For more information about Peanut Allergy:

American Academy of Asthma, Allergy & Immunology 611 E. Wells Street Milwaukee, WI 53202-3889 414.272.6071	American College of Allergy, Asthma, and Immunology 85 West Algonquin Road Arlington Heights, IL 60005
American Allergy Association P.O. Box 7273 Menlo Park, CA 94026 415.322.1663	Food Allergy Network 10400 Eaton Place, Suite 107 Fairfax, VA 22030 800.929.4040; 703.691.3179 www.foodallergy.org www.fankids.org (for kids)
American Dietetic Association 216 W. Jackson Boulevard Chicago, IL 60606-6995 800.745.0775 ext. 5000 http://www.eatright.org	

Note: Be sure to check with your health professional about peanut-free diets.

Soy-Sensitivity Fact Sheet
Food Allergy Field Guide (Savory Palate, 2000)
by Theresa Willingham

Symptoms of sensitivity to soy products include skin rashes, gastrointestinal problems, facial swelling, shortness of breath, difficulty swallowing, and possibly even anaphylactic reaction.

At least 15 different allergenic proteins have been found in soy. Soy sensitivity seems largely dependent on how the soy is processed. Fermented soy products like miso and tofu typically cause less sensitivity problems than raw soybeans. Because soy is an inexpensive, high protein food, it is used as a base for many different prepared foods

Even though some soy products may not cause a reaction, it's best to avoid all soy because it's difficult to evaluate the level of processing or safety of the food. This includes anything with hydrolyzed vegetable protein, textured soy protein, tofu, miso, natto, okara, soy cheese, soy sauces, soy protein concentrates, isolates and flours, tempeh, soy beverages, yuba, and soy lecithin. Mono and digylcerides, as well as mono-sodium glutamate may contain soy. Soy oil contains no proteins so should be safe (unless it's cold-pressed). If unsure, avoid it.

⊘ AVOID	☑ OK
Hydrolyzed vegetable protein.	*Use only vegetable proteins whose source is identified.*
Lecithin.	*Avoid.*
Miso.	*Avoid.*
Mono-diglyceride.	*Check for exact source or avoid.*
Monosodium glutamate.	*Ask manufacturer about source.*
Natural flavors.	*Know exact source.*
Soy cheese, a substitute for sour cream or cream cheese, is soy.	*Regular cheeses, sour cream or cream cheese.*
Soy fiber (okara, soy bran, and soy isolate) can be food ingredient.	*Oat or other grain fiber.*
Soy flour.	*Oat, wheat, rice, or other flours.*
Soy grits.	*Corn grits.*
Soy meal and soy oil are used in inks, soaps, and cosmetics.	*Check manufacturer for specifics.*

⊘ AVOID	☑ OK
Soy milk, and its derivatives like soy yogurt.	Regular milk, goats milk, etc. and their derivatives.
Soy oil. (cold-pressed)	100% pure canola, olive, peanut, safflower, or other OK oils.
Natto, Tofu, Tempeh, Soy protein, Soy sauces (shoyu, tamari, soya)	Avoid.
Vegetable oil	Know source, ask manufacturer.
Vegetable protein.	Know source, ask manufacturer.
Vitamin E.	Use Cod Liver Oil or soy-free E

Additional words that *may* denote soy include: bean flour, edamame beans, miso, vegetable protein concentrate, hydrolyzed plant protein (HPP), hydrolyzed soy protein, hydrolyzed vegetable protein (HVP), lectin, soy lecithin, texturized vegetable protein (TVP), vegetable broth, vegetable gum, and vegetable starch.

For more information about Soy Sensitivity:

American Allergy Association P.O. Box 7273 Menlo Park, CA 94026 415.322.1663	American Academy of Asthma, Allergy, & Immunology 611 E. Wells Street Milwaukee, WI 53202-3889 414.272.6071
American College of Allergy, Asthma, and Immunology 85 West Algonquin Road Arlington Heights, IL 60005	Food Allergy Network 10400 Eaton Place, Suite 107 Fairfax, VA 22030 800.929.4040; 703.691.3179 www.foodallergy.org www.fankids.org (for kids)
American Dietetic Association 216 W. Jackson Boulevard Chicago, IL 60606-6995 800.745.0775 ext. 5000 http://www.eatright.org	

Note: Be sure to check with your health professional about soy-free diets.

Wheat-Sensitivity Fact Sheet
Food Allergy Field Guide (Savory Palate, 2000)
by Theresa Willingham

Wheat sensitivities can result from an inability to digest the various proteins in wheat. Celiac disease, one of the most common of the wheat sensitivities, results from an inability to digest gluten proteins. Technically, it is an autoimmune disorder wherein the immune system reacts to gluten by damaging the villi, the little fingerlike projections that line the small intestine and aid in the absorption of nutrients. This can lead to malnutrition and other problems.

Gluten proteins are found in members of the grass family of wheat, barley, rye, and triticale, and occur in their derivatives, as well. Things like malt, grain starches, hydrolyzed vegetable/plant proteins, textured vegetable proteins, grain vinegars, soy sauce, grain alcohol, flavorings, and many of the binders and fillers found in vitamins and medications contain gluten and can trigger the autoimmune response in sensitive individuals. The only treatment for celiac disease and other wheat sensitivities is a diet free of wheat, barley, oats (largely due to the danger of cross-contamination from shared processing facilities—in and of themselves, they do not contain gluten), and rye.

⃠ AVOID	☑ OK
Calcium caseinate or Sodium caseinate (contains MSG).	Calcium phosphate, calcium chloride.
Dextrins.	Maltodextrin (made from corn)
Hydrolyzed vegetable protein.	Know exact source.
Hydrolyzed plant protein.	Know exact source.
Malt.	Maltodextrin.
Modified food starch.	Know exact source, e.g., potato.

⊘ AVOID	☑ OK
Mono and di-glycerides.	*Know exact source.*
Rice malt (can contain barley or Koji).	*Rice or other flour, without malt.*

Avoid these grain products:		**Vary the use of these:**	
Barley	*Graham*	*Bean flours*	*Potato flour*
Bulgur	*Kamut*	*Corn flour*	*Potato starch*
Bran	*Orzo*	*Corn meal*	*Rice flour*
Couscous	*Rye*	*Corn starch*	*Soy flour*
Durum	*Semolina*	*Nut flours*	*Tapioca flour*
Einkorn	*Spelt*		
Farina	*Triticale*		

For more information about wheat sensitivities:

American Academy of Asthma, Allergy, & Immunology 611 E. Wells Street Milwaukee, WI 53202-3889 414.272.6071	American Dietetic Association 216 W. Jackson Boulevard Chicago, IL 60606-6995 800.745.0775 ext. 5000 http://www.eatright.org
American College of Allergy, Asthma, and Immunology 85 West Algonquin Road Arlington Heights, IL 60005	Celiac Disease Foundation 13251 Ventura Boulevard, Suite 1 Studio City, CA 91604-1838 (818) 990-2379; 818.990.2379 - fax www.celiac.org/cdf
Celiac Sprue Association/United States of America, Inc. P.O. Box 31700 Omaha, NE 68131-0700 402.558.0600 www.csaceliacs.org	Food Allergy Network 10400 Eaton Place, Suite 107 Fairfax, VA 22030 800.929.4040; 703.691.3179 www.foodallergy.org www.fankids.org (for kids)
Gluten Intolerance Group of North America P.O. Box 23053 Seattle, WA 98102-0353 (206) 325-6980 gig@accessone.com www.gluten.net	National Digestive Diseases Information Clearinghouse 2 Information Way Bethesda, MD 20892-3570 301.6543810

Note: Be sure to check with your health professional about wheat/free-gluten/free diets.

251

Food Families

Understanding which foods belong to which food families can help you plan rotation style diets better, and possibly predict—or at least better understand—some cross reactions to various foods.

The charts below are not comprehensive, but they do feature the most common foods we eat and to which we may develop sensitivities. The majority of the information on these lists was compiled from Dr. Harris Steinman's FAP AID food analysis program.

Legumes

Acacia	*Karaya gum*	*Soybean*
Acacia gum	*Kidney bean*	*Soybean oil*
Alfalfa	*Lentil*	*Soybean flour*
Arabic	*Licorice*	*Soybean lecithin*
Black-eyed pea	*Lima bean*	*Split pea*
Carob	*Locust bean gum*	*String bean*
Carob (St. John's	*Mung bean*	*Talca gum*
Bread)	*Navy*	*Tamarind*
Cassia chick pea	*Peanut*	*Tonka bean*
Field pea	*Peanut oil*	*Tragancanth gum*
Green bean	*Pinto bean*	*Urid flour*
Green Pea		

Citrus

Angostura	*Grapefruit*	*Lime*
Citrange	*Kumquat*	*Orange*
Citron	*Lemon*	*Tangerine*

Cereals

Bamboo Shoots	*Corn oil*	*Patent*
Barley	*Corn starch*	*Flour (wheat)*
Barley, Malt*	*Corn sugar*	*Oats*
Bran (wheat)	*Corn syrup*	*Rice*
Cane sugar	*Corn dextrose*	*Rye**
Cane molasses	*Corn glucose*	*Sorghum*
Chestnut, Water	*Corn cerelose*	*Triticale*
Chestnut, Ling nut	*Farina (wheat)*	*Wheat*
Chestnut, Singhara nut	*Graham flour (wheat)*	*Wheat flour*
Corn	*Gluten flour (wheat)*	*Wheat germ*
Corn meal	*Millet*	*Wheat (whole) flour*
		Wild rice

Nightshade

Brinjal	Bell pepper	Pimento
Cayenne	Chili pepper	Potato
Capsicum	Green pepper	Tabasco
Eggplant	Red pepper	Thorn apple
Ground cherry	Sweet pepper	Tobacco
Banana pepper	Paprika	Tomato

Mustard

Broccoli	Collard	Mustard
Brussels sprouts	Colza shoots	Mustard greens
Cabbage	Kale	Radish
Cauliflower	Kohlrabi	Rutabaga
Celery cabbage	Kraut	Turnips
Chinese cabbage	Horseradish	Watercress

Carrot/Parsley

Anise/Aniseed	Coriander/Cilantro/Italian parsley	Fennel
Caraway		Parsley
Carrot	Cumin	Parsnip
Celery	Dill	

Rose/Apple

Apple	Crab-apple	Plum
Apple cider/vinegar	Damson plum	Prune
Apple pectin	Loganberry	Quince
Apricot	Loquat	Raspberry
Blackberry	Nectarine	Rosehip
Boysenberry	Peach	Salmon berry
Cherry	Pear	Strawberry

Composite Family/Aster

Absinthe	Endive	Sunflower & Seeds
Artichoke	Escarole	Sunflower Oil
Artichoke, Jerusalem	Head lettuce	Vermouth
Chamomile	Lettuce	Vermouth (Ragweed)
Celtuse	Leaf lettuce	Vermouth
Chicory	Oyster plant, Salsify	Pyrethrum
Dandelion	Sesame seed oil	Yarrow

Lily

Aloe	Hyacinth	Sarsaparilla
Asparagus	Leek	Scallion
Chives	Onion	Shallot
Garlic		

Walnut

Black walnut	English walnut	Pecan
Butternut	Hickory nut	

Mint

Basil	Lemon balm	Rosemary
Bergamot	Marjoram	Sage
Horehound	Mint	Savory
Hyssop	Oregano	Spearmint
Lavender	Peppermint	Thyme

These are just some of the larger food families, in which sensitivities to various members of the food families may develop. There are many smaller families, with only one or two members, to which sensitivities may also develop. These include, but are not limited to:

- Birch family: filbert, hazelnut, wintergreen
- Brazil nut
- Beech: beechnut and chestnut
- Cashew: cashew, mango, pistachio
- Heath: blueberry, cranberry, huckleberry
- Pineapple
- Yam: Includes sweet potato (one of the least allergenic foods)

And there are some hard to classify, but useful foods in which sensitivities are rare, including:

- Quinoa: (*Chenopodium quinoa Willdenow,* a member of the goosefoot family) which is used as cereal crop, but is not a grass. It is related to lamb's quarters and classified as a *pseudocereal*[151]
- Amaranth: (*Amaranthus,* a member of the *Caryophyllales family*) a "potherb," not a grass. One of 60 species in this annual. It is sometimes known as pigweed.
- Buckwheat: Not a grass, but an herb in the family *polygonum.* It is related to rhubarb.

And there are also the edible members of the mammal family, bird family (egg sensitivity would fall under this family), fish, and shell-fish families—the latter two containing several members to which many people have sensitivities.

---

* See Johnson, D. L., and S.M. Ward, Quinoa, p. 219-221, in J. Janek and J.E. Simon (eds) New Crops, Wiley, NY, 1993. For more information on quinoa, amaranth, and buckwheat, see The Splendid Grain by Rebecca Wood, William Morrow, NY 1999

Nutrition Facts
Meals that Count

It's important, whether you're fixing meals for your child at home or eating out, to make sure your child (and everyone else in the family!) is eating a healthy, well-rounded diet. We've already discussed how easy it is to slip into a dietary rut when dealing with food sensitivities. But besides culinary boredom, an unvaried diet may result in poor nutrition.

Nutrition from the Ground Up
The traditional food pyramid most of us are familiar with is the brainchild of the USDA. It is fair to say the USDA has our best interests at heart with its design.

The Food Pyramid

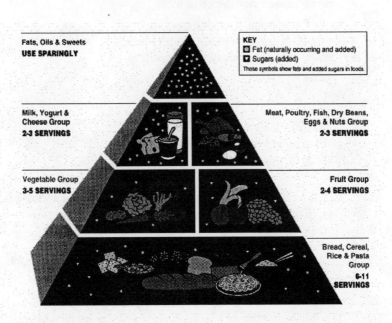

It's recommended that two to six year olds, for instance, should eat six servings a day from the grain group (assuming a 1600 calorie daily diet), while older children, teenaged girls, active

255

women and most men should consume nine servings (based on a 2200 calorie a day diet). Teenaged boys and active men, say the guidelines, should eat 11 servings from the grain group.

The recommendations in the food pyramid and in the USDA's Dietary Guidelines reflect just plain common sense, and therefore seem as good a place as any to start when planning a good, healthy diet.[152]

The USDA[153] describes servings as follows, starting at the bottom of the pyramid and working up:

☑ For the Bread, Cereal, Rice and Pasta Group (grains), a serving can consist of any of the following:
- 1 slice of bread
- About 1 cup of ready-to-eat cereal flakes
- ½ cup cooked cereal, rice or pasta

☑ In the Fruit Group, a serving can consist of:
- 1 medium apple, banana, orange or pear
- ½ cup chopped, cooked, or canned fruit
- ¾ cup of fruit juice

☑ In the Vegetable Group, a serving can be:
- 1 cup raw leafy vegetables
- ½ cup other vegetables cooked or raw
- ¾ cup of vegetable juice

☑ In the Milk, Yogurt, and Cheese Group (Dairy) a serving is:
- 1 cup of milk or yogurt (including lactose-free and lactose-reduced dairy products)
- 1 ½ ounces natural cheese, like cheddar
- 2 ounces processed cheese, like American
- 1 cup soy-based beverage with added calcium

---

[152] According to the American Dietetic Association, recommendations call for children to increase their fruit and vegetable consumption to 5 or more servings daily. The ADA says that the qualitative guidelines put forth in the Dietary Guidelines for Americans and the Food Guide Pyramid is an excellent tool for educating consumers on how to achieve the dietary recommendations.
[153] All the USDA information in this discussion reflects the most recent updates (March 2000) by the USDA Dietary Guidelines Council.

☑ In the Meat, Poultry, Fish, Dry Beans, Eggs and Nuts Group (Meat and Beans Group)
- 2-3 ounces cooked lean meat, poultry or fish
- ½ cup of cooked dry beans (dry beans, peas, and lentils can be counted as servings in either the meat and beans group or the vegetable group. As a vegetable, ½ cup beans counts as 1 serving. As a meat substitute, 1 cup of beans is 1 serving).
- ½ cup tofu counts as 1 ounce of lean meat
- 2 ½ ounce soy burger or 1 egg counts as 1 ounce of lean meat
- 2 tablespoons of peanut butter or 1/3 cup of nuts counts as 1 ounce of meat.

The USDA does note—without comment—that these serving sizes are smaller than those on the Nutrition Facts labels. It uses the example of 1 serving of cooked cereal, rice or pasta as being 1 cup for the label, but only ½ cup for the pyramid. Obviously, that's why these are called "guidelines." The point is, they are fairly reasonable ones. And very modern ones. These serving suggestions reflect the Dietary Guidelines Advisory Committee's most recent efforts to take into account dietary differences that may exist for a variety of reasons.

"Different people like different foods and like to prepare the same foods in different ways," the Committee acknowledges in its year 2000 update. "Culture, family background, religion, moral beliefs, the cost and availability of food, life experiences, food intolerances and allergies affect people's food choices." The Pyramid, it says, should be considered a "starting point to shape your eating patterns."

And clearly, the inclusion of such food items as tofu and soy burgers speaks to that acknowledgement. But the USDA doesn't have the only pyramid in town. The food pyramid concept can been used to describe the eating styles of many cultures. Some of these can be quite helpful in managing a special diet, if only because it helps us make that paradigm shift away from the traditional American diet.

An Asian food pyramid,[154] for example, has grains at its foundation, too, headed up by rice, millet, and corn. Above the grains are fruits,

---

[154] All ethnic food pyramid discussions are derived from Oldways Preservation and Exchange Diet, a non-profit organization whose mission is to "encourage healthy eating by promoting sustainable food choices and traditional, wonderful foods of many cultures. Contact Oldways

257

legumes, nuts, seeds, and vegetables. Vegetable oils are actually considered part of the pyramid and precede fish, shellfish, and dairy products. Above those are eggs and poultry, then sweets—followed by meats at the very top. A Mediterranean food pyramid would also be based on daily servings of grains, including couscous, polenta, and potatoes. That would be followed by daily servings of fruits, beans, legumes, nuts and vegetables. Olive oil follows those (also considered an essential part of the pyramid here), then cheese and yogurt, followed by fish, poultry, eggs, and sweets, each eaten a few times a week. At the very top of that pyramid would be red meat.

But generally, most good diets are based on the sane and safe principal that the more grains, fruits, and vegetables you eat, the healthier you will be. The USDA's Dietary Guidelines for Americans focuses on seven principals, of which the 7th, drinking alcoholic beverages in moderation, shouldn't apply to your child. The other six, however, are valuable and worth reviewing briefly, with an eye to how food sensitivities actually necessitate adherence to most of these healthy guidelines:

☑ *Eat a Variety of Foods*. No single food can supply all the nutrients in the amounts you need, nutritional experts point out. Milk (or an appropriate substitute), for example, supplies calcium but little iron. Meat supplies iron but little calcium. Variety equals nutrition. *Just being food sensitive requires your child eat a variety of foods, so you can check this one off right from the get-go!*

☑ *Maintain Healthy Weight.* If you or your child is too fat or too thin, you are more likely to develop health problems. Eating properly helps maintain a healthy weight. *Being overweight is rarely a problem for the food sensitive and if your child sticks to his or her prescribed diet, a good healthy weight should follow.*

☑ *Choose a Diet Low in Fat, Saturated Fat, and Cholesterol. This is usually the food sensitive child's birthright. Most of the alternative foods they eat are low in all these fats, whereas the majority of Americans have diets high in fat, saturated fat, and cholesterol.* Such diets are linked to increased risk for heart disease, obesity, and certain types of cancer. The USDA sets the following goals for fat and saturated fats in

---

Preservation and Exchange Trust at 25 First St., Cambridge, MA 02141; phone 617-621-3000 or email oldways@tiac.net. <http://www.oldwayspt.org/html/pyramid.htm>

258

American diets. Remember that these goals for fats *apply to the diet over several days, not to a single meal or food.*

☑ **Total Fat.** Your goal for fat depends on your calorie needs. An amount that provides 30 percent or less of calories is suggested.

☑ **Saturated Fat.** An amount that provides less than 10 percent of calories is suggested. All fats contain both saturated and unsaturated fat (fatty acids). Animal products are the main sources of saturated fat in most diets, with tropical oils (coconut, palm kernel, and palm oils) and hydrogenated fats providing smaller amounts. Strive for less hydrogenated fat in your diet.

☑ **Cholesterol.** Animal products are the sources of all dietary cholesterol. Eating less fat from animal sources will help lower the cholesterol, total fat, and saturated fat in your diet.

☑ *Choose A Diet with Plenty of Vegetables, Fruits and Grain Products.* A varied diet of vegetables, including dry beans and peas; fruits; and breads, cereals, pasta, and rice supplies important vitamins and minerals, fiber, and complex carbohydrates—and is generally lower in fat. It's better to get fiber from foods that contain fiber naturally rather than from supplements. Some of the benefit from a high fiber diet may be from the food that provides the fiber, not from fiber alone. *Again, this one typically comes with the territory.*

☑ *Use Sugars Only in Moderation* Sugars and many foods that contain them in large amounts supply calories but are limited in nutrients. Sugar comes in many forms, such as table sugar (sucrose), brown sugar, honey, syrup, corn sweetener, high-fructose corn sweetener, molasses, glucose (dextrose), fructose, maltose and lactose. *We would all do well to heed this advice, because it's easy for even the food sensitive to overuse sugar.*

☑ *Use Salt and Sodium Only in Moderation.* Most Americans eat more salt and sodium than they need. In populations with diets low in salt, high blood pressure is less common than in populations with saltier diets. Eating less salt and sodium will benefit those people whose blood pressure goes up with salt intake. *Same as above. Too much salt isn't good for children or adults.*

259

In its year 2000 recommendations, the USDA renewed its emphasis on activity as well, recommending less sedentary behavior, especially for children. Their new proposed changes focus on an ABC of good health that 1) Aims for fitness, 2) Builds a healthy base, and 3) Encourages Americans to choose their foods sensibly.[155]

Everyone can meet all of these guidelines and recommendations fairly easily, even if they can't tolerate certain grains, fruits, vegetables, or dairy products.

Supplement Facts: Nutrient Stealers

Early in our research we learned that, by virtue of being wheat sensitive, Chris had a tendency to be deficient in certain nutrients. In fact, food sensitivities of any kind can be nutrient stealers. Undiagnosed, the body's inability to digest wheat, milk, peanut, egg and soy proteins, or certain sugars triggers digestive disorders lessen absorption of the right nutrients in the proper amounts.

For those who are sensitive to several foods, there is the problem of simply not being able to eat the right foods, or the proper combinations of foods, that produce good health. Even if you're familiar with all the proper exchanges and substitutes, if your child is sensitive to corn, wheat, eggs, and milk, it makes it a little harder to get the right nutrients in the right amounts. And that's where supplements can come in handy, just to hedge your nutritional bets—and your child's health—a little.

What Every Child Needs

Just as the USDA sets guidelines for healthy eating, it makes recommendations for safe and adequate nutritional supplementation. Here's what the USDA suggests your children, from newborn to age 10, should have:

Age (Yr)	0-6 mo.	6 mo.-1 yr	1-3	4-6	7-10
(Kg)	6	9	13	20	28
(Lb)	13	20	29	44	62
(Cm)	60	71	90	112	132
(Inches)	24	28	35	44	52
Kcal (Energy)	650	850	1300	1800	2000
(G) Protein	13	14	16	24	28

---

[155] The Dietary Guidelines Advisory Committee

260

(Ug RE) Vitamin A	375	375	400	500	700
(Ug) Vitamin D	7.5	10	10	10	10
(Mg A-TE) Vit E	3	4	6	7	7
(Ug) Vit K	5	10	15	20	30
(Mg) Vit C	30	35	40	45	45
(Mg) Thiamin	0.3	0.4	0.7	0.9	1
(Mg) Riboflavin	0.4	0.5	0.8	1.1	1.2
(Mg NE) Niacin	5	6	9	12	13
(Mg) Vit B6	0.3	0.6	1	1.1	1.4
(Ug) Folate	25	35	50	75	100
(Ug) Vit B12	0.3	0.5	0.7	1	1.4
(Mg) Calcium	400	600	800	800	800
(Mg) Phosphorus	300	500	800	800	800
(Mg) Magnesium	40	60	80	120	170
(Mg) Iron	6	10	10	10	10
(Mg) Zinc	5	5	10	10	10
(Ug) Iodine	40	50	70	90	120
(Ug) Selenium	10	15	20	20	30

It's important to remember that nutrients from foods come with many additional benefits that vitamin and mineral supplements can't replicate alone. Vitamins don't replace good food. In fact, they aren't assimilated without eating other food with them. That's why it's usually suggested that vitamins be taken with meals. Here's a brief look at the principal vitamins and minerals in our diets.

Vitamin ABCs

Vitamins* regulate our metabolism and help convert food to energy. They are considered "micronutrients" because the body needs them in relatively small amounts compared to things like carbohydrates, proteins, fats, and water. Here are a few of the most import-ant vitamins our bodies need and how our bodies use them.[156]

Vitamin	Necessary For
Vitamin A (Beta carotene)	Protects against night-blindness and air pollutants; counter-acts weak eyesight; for skin, as in acne.
Thiamine (Vitamin B1)	Essential for functioning of nervous system, muscles, heart; stabilizes appetite; promotes growth & good muscle tone.
Riboflavin (Vitamin B2)	Metabolizes carbohydrate, fat & protein; aids in forming antibodies and red blood cells, maintains cell respiration; necessary for maintenance of vision, skin, nails, and hair. Alleviates eye fatigue; promotes general health.
Niacin (Vitamin B3)	Improves circulation; reduces cholesterol level in blood; maintains nervous system; helps maintain healthy skin, tongue, and digestion.
Pantothenic Acid (Vitamin B5)	Releases energy from carbohydrates, fats, and protein; aids utilization of vitamins; improves immune system and resistance to stress; helps cell building, development of central nervous system, and adrenal glands. Allergies.
Biotin	Utilizes protein, folic acid, pantothenic acid, and vitamin B-12, promotes healthy hair.
Vitamin C	Healthy teeth, gums, bones; helps heal wounds, scar tissue, fractures; prevents scurvy, builds resistance to infection; aids prevention and treatment of common cold.
Vitamin D	Absorption, utilization of calcium and phosphorus; vital to normal growth/development of bones and teeth in children.
Vitamin E	Promotes healthy skin and hair, necessary for tissue repair, maintains healthy nerves and muscle.

*Vitamins can be oil or water soluble. Oil soluble vitamins can be stored for long periods of time in fatty tissue and the liver and include vitamins A, D, E, and K. Water soluble vitamins aren't stored by the body, but excreted in body fluids within four days, so they need to be ingested daily.

---

[156] For more complete vitamin information, contact the USDA.

262

Mineral Ps & Qs

Minerals are naturally-occurring elements found in the earth. Every living thing on earth requires them for healthy functioning. In humans, minerals balance our body fluids, help in the formation of blood, bone, and proper nerve function, regulate muscle tone, and maintain a proper balance of chemicals in our bodies. They're stored mostly in bone and muscle tissue.

Mineral	Important For
Calcium	Strong bones, teeth, healthy gums; regulates heartbeat, nerve impulse transmission, proper bone growth and bone mineral density in children, proper blood clotting, healthy skin, cells, energy.
Copper	Aids formation of bone, hemoglobin, and red blood cells; works with zinc and Vitamin C to form elastin; formation of collagen, helps healing processes, energy production; also needed for healthy nerves and joints.
Iodine	Metabolizes excess fat, important for physical and mental development, and healthy thyroid functioning.
Iron	Production of hemoglobin and myoglobin (hemoglobin in muscle tissue) and oxygenation of red blood cells.
Magnesium	Important in enzyme activity; assists calcium and potassium uptake; prevents calcification of soft tissue; strengthens arterial linings, helps formation of bone; metabolizes carbohydrate and minerals.
Phosphorous	Necessary for healthy bones, teeth; cell growth; healthy heart and kidney function; assists utilization of vitamins and converting food to energy.
Potassium	Healthy nervous system, regular heart rhythm, proper muscle function; controls body's water balance; controls and maintains proper cell chemical reactions and transfer of nutrients through cell membranes.
Sodium	Maintains body's water balance and blood pH, and for nerve, stomach, and muscle function.
Zinc	Helps maintain healthy immune system, proper healing.

Using Supplements Safely

Obviously, your child's doctor, dietitian, or nutritionist will be your best guide in establishing a good vitamin and mineral regime for your child. What is clear, though, is that children with food sensitivities can benefit from supplements, typically at half the adult dosages recommended by the manufacturer, or according to the DRI for

263

children. Also, keep in mind that *whatever supplements you choose for your child must be free of allergens that cause the food sensitivity* in the first place.

That means you have to read supplement labels as carefully as you read any other labels. The FDA has requirements of supplement manufacturers as the USDA does of food manufacturers, and all supplements produced in the U.S. must have the following information on the label:

- Statement of identity (e.g., "ginseng")
- Net quantity of contents (e.g., "60 capsules")
- Structure-function claim and the statement "This statement has not been evaluated by the Food and Drug Administration. This product is not intended to diagnose, treat, cure, or prevent any disease."
- Directions for use (e.g., "Take one capsule daily.")
- Supplement Facts panel (lists serving size, amount, and active ingredient)
- Other ingredients in descending order of predominance and by common name or proprietary blend.
- Name and place of business of manufacturer, packer or distributor. This is the address to write for more product information.

Be sure to read the ingredients listing carefully, and if you're in doubt about any item, call the manufacturer. Remember, you can find allergen-free vitamins in most health food stores, or use the resources mentioned in the back of the book to locate additional allergen-free vitamin suppliers.

Who Needs What

For the *cow-milk-allergic and gluten intolerant*, consider [157] :

👍 *A good allergen-free children's multi-vitamin formulation* that includes: B complex, calcium, magnesium, and vitamins C and E.

👍 *Digestive Enzymes,* which aid in the breakdown and absorption of foods. Check with your doctor or nutritionist to see if these are appropriate for your child.

👍 *Acidophilus Fiber* supplements may improve fiber intake.

For those with *peanut, egg, corn, and soy sensitivities*, those supplements plus extra:

👍 *Potassium*, to assist the adrenal glands.

👍 *Zinc*, for improved immune system function.

👍 *Manganese*, in chelated form, to help the body's enzyme system.

The Enzyme Factor

Although not all experts agree, it's been suggested that those with food intolerances or sensitivities tend to be deficient in three possible enzymes[158] that help keep the body detoxified. Enzymes are protein molecules that act as catalysts in almost all the body's biochemical activities and are essential for digestion, brain activity, and healthy cell function.

Enzymes are divided into two types, digestive and metabolic, and each has specific functions. Enzymes also help "detoxify" the foods we eat, which, if not broken down into forms our bodies can use, can sometimes act as poisons. In one respect, that's what your children's bodies are reacting to when their bodies don't digest proteins, sugars,

---

[157] Compiled from the Allergy Connection (website address in back) and Balch, James F., M.D. and Phyllis A. Balch, Prescription for Nutritional Healing, New York: Avery Publishing Group, 1997.
[158] From "The Physicians Handbook for Clinical Nutrition," <www.moreton.com.au/ana/inform>.

or other portions of food properly. The enzymes those with food intolerances seem to lack are:

- *Phenol Suphotransferase*, which detoxifies phenols in the body. It is thought to be activated by artificial food colorings.
- *Mono-Amine Oxidase*, which reduces the chemicals tyramine and phenylethylamine in the body—which may cause rebound headaches.
- *Enzymes that oxidize sulphide chemicals to less harmful sulphoxide.* As much as 80% of those with food intolerances are deficient in these enzymes.

Consequently, it might be helpful to supplement the diet of those with sensitivities to peanut, eggs, soy, and corn with digestive enzymes, in addition to vitamin and mineral supplements. Again, you'll need to talk to your child's doctor or nutritionist to determine whether enzyme are right for your child. But for maximum effectiveness, the enzyme you choose should contain all three enzyme groups: amylase, pro-tease, and lipase. Digestive enzymes are best taken after meals.

Another digestive problem that might be at issue in malabsorption problems is hypochlorydria, or hydrochloric acid (HCL) deficiency. Possibly as many as 80% of patients with food sensitivities suffer from some degree of this deficiency. Those with inadequate HCL secretion may not properly digest proteins, vitamins, and minerals. Symptoms include heartburn, passage of undigested food in the stool, anemia and other mineral deficiencies, and yeast infections.

Treatment of hypochlorhydria consists of supplementing the diet with hydrochloric acid—either betaine HCL from beets, or glutamic HCL from grains. Either type of supplementation should be done under medical supervision, as HCL can damage the stomach lining if taken in excessive doses. Again, talk to your doctor about this.

Supplement, Don't Replace!
These are just a few possibilities to help give your child's body a boost in recovering from a food sensitivity and a nudge in the right direction as you embark on his or her healthy new diet. Remember, though, that supplements are just that—vitamin and mineral assists taken in addition to a good healthy diet of the appropriate fruits,

266

vegetables, grains, and other foods. Supplements are not a replacement for food, and can only work hand in hand with a good diet.

The best things you can do to maximize your own and your child's health are[159]:

👍 **Eat Natural Foods**, minimally processed and in as close to their natural state as possible. Foods altered with additives, salt, sugar, and fats tend to be deficient in the nutrients we need for maximum health.

👍 **Eat a Varied Diet,** consisting of a wide variety of foods. This not only reduces the chances for additional sensitivities, but also provides a greater range from which to obtain nutrients.

👍 **Eat Small, Frequent Meals** instead of large meals three times a day. "Nibbling" is traditionally better than gorging, allowing food to digest more adequately, providing a more stable blood sugar level throughout the day, and lowering risks of heart disease, diabetes, and obesity.

👍 **Eat nutrient-dense foods, like** fresh vegetables, whole grains, legumes, and fruit, and low fat meats (turkey, fish, and chicken).

👍 **Focus on quality of weight**, instead of quantity of weight. Your aim should be for a reasonable percent of body fat in your child, rather than a particular weight. The USDA BMI (Body Mass Index) is a good indicator of reasonable body fat. To discover you or your child's BMI, multiply weight (in pounds) by 703, multiply height (in inches) by height (in inches), and divide the first answer by the second answer to get your BMI. A BMI of between 19 and 25 or 26 is considered healthy.

👍 **Eat enough protein,** on average 1-2 grams of protein for each kilogram of body weight. Example: 150 pound patient. Divide 150 pounds by 2.2 to find 68 kilograms, multiply by 1 to 2, yields 68-136 grams of protein daily for a healthy immune system.

---

[159] Adapted from "Laws of Nutrition," by Patrick Quillin, Ph.D., R.D., C.N.S.

267

👍 **Use supplements in addition to**, rather than instead of, good food. The best place to get vitamins and minerals is from the food you eat.

Government Agencies

Food & Drug Administration	U.S. Department of Agriculture
Office of Consumer Affairs 5600 Fishers Lane, HFE 88 Rockville, MD 20857 800.FDA.4010; 301.827.4420 http://www.fda.gov/	14th & Independence Ave., SW Washington, D.C. 20250 202.720.2791 http://www.usda.gov/usda.htm

National Institutes of Health (NIH)
Bethesda, MD 20892 Contact at: National Digestive Diseases Information Clearinghouse 301.654.3810 http://www.nih.gov/

Dining and Travel Clubs

Sully's Living Without magazine, *a lifestyle guide for people with food and/or chemical sensitivities.*	Bob & Ruth's Gluten-Free Dining & Travel Club.
PO Box 46 Glencoe, IL 60022-0046 630.415.3378 www.livingwithout.com Upscale gluten-free adventures.	22 Breton Hill Rd., Suite 1B, Pikesville, MD 21208 410.486.0292 bobolevy@juno.com Gluten-free travel and newsletter.

Resources and Associations
This list is not complete. Please verify all information before using.

Allergies, Asthma, and Anaphylaxis

American Academy of Allergy, Asthma, & Immunology 611 E. Wells Street Milwaukee, WI 53202-3889 414.272.6071 www.aaaai.org	Allergy and Asthma Network/ Mothers of Asthmatics 3554 Chain Bridge Road, Suite 200 Fairfax, VA 22030-2709 800-822-2762 www.aanma.org
American Dietetic Association 216 W. Jackson Boulevard Chicago, IL 60606-6995 800.745.0775 ext. 5000 http://www.eatright.org	American College of Allergy, Asthma, and Immunology 85 West Algonquin Road Arlington Heights, IL 60005 http://allergy.mcg.edu
Anaphylaxis Campaign P.O. Box 149 Fleet, Hampshire, UK GUI39XU www.anaphylaxis.org	Asthma & Allergy Foundation .of America 1233 20th Street, N.W., Suite 402 Washington, DC 20036 202.466.7643; 202.466.8940 fax 800-7ASTHMA; www.aafa.org
Food Allergy Network 10400 Eaton Place, Suite 107 Fairfax, VA 22030 800.9294040; 703.6913179 www.foodallergy.org www.fankids.org (for kids)	International Food Information Council 1100 Connecticut Ave. NW #430 Washington, D.C. 20036 http://ificinfo.health.org/ e-mail: foodinfo@ificinfo.health.org
Medic Alert® Foundation 800.432.5378 $35 initial registration fee; $15/yearly Hypoallergenic versions available	PeanutAllergy.Com 123 Grant Ave Medford, MA 02155 781.395.9530; 603.388.5483 fax e-mail: Contact@PeanutAllergy.Com http://www.peanutallergy.com/index.htm
Bullseye Information Services 200 Linden Street, Dept. 1A Wellesley, MA 02181 508.647.0938	La Leche League International 1400 N. Meacham Road P.O. Box 4079 Schaumburg, IL 60168-4079 800.LALECHE

269

Celiac Sprue

Celiac Sprue Assn/USA, Inc. P.O. Box 31700 Omaha, NE 68131-0700 402.558.0600 www.csaceliacs.org	Gluten Intolerance Group of NA (GIG) ~~PO Box 23053~~ 11015 10th Ave SW, Suite A Seattle, WA ~~98102-0353~~ 98166 206.~~325.6980~~ 2466652 gig@accessone.com; www.gig.net
National Digestive Disease Infor.Clearinghouse 2 Information Way Bethesda, MD 20892-3570 301.654.3810	Tri-County Celiac Sprue Group 34638 Beechwood St. Farmington Hills, MI 48335 (Tri-Counties Shopping List - $10))

Autism

Autism Society of America 7910 Woodmont Avenue, Suite 300 Bethesda, MD 20814-3015 800.3AUTISM, extension 150 or 301.657.0881; 301.657.0869 fax	Autism Network for Dietary Intervention (ANDI) P.O. Box 17711 Rochester, NY 14617-0711 609.737.8453 fax http://members.aol.com/autismndi/ PAGES/index.htm
Center for the Study of Autism P.O. Box 4538 Salem, OR 97302 www.autism.org	Cure Autism Now 5225 Wilshire Boulevard, Suite 226 Los Angeles, CA 90036 323.549.0500 1-888-8AUTISM email info@cureautismnow.org www.canfoundation.org

ADHD and Other Behavioral Or Learning Disorders

Feingold Association of the U.S. P.O. Box 6550 Alexandria, VA 22306 800.321.3287 www.feingold.org	National Attention Deficit Disorder Assn. 1788 Second Street, Suite 200 Highland Park, IL 60035 847.432.2332 www.add.org

270

Software

NuConnexions (Diet & Nutrition) P.O. Box 269, Queensville, ON, L0G 1R0, Canada 905.478-8915; 905.478.8916 - fax e-mail (info@nuconnexions.com) http://www.nuconnexions.com/	NutriGenie P. O. Box 8226 Stanford, CA 94309 e-mail: NutriGenie@aol.com or http://pages.prodigy.com/CA/nutrige nie/websites.html
Dr. Harris Steinman, FAP AID, Zing Solutions P.O. Box 565, Milnerton 7435, South Africa tel/fax +27(0)21.551.2993 http://zingsolutions.com/food/ (Regular price is $200; $160 For *Food Allergy Field Guide* readers)	

Online Resources (We assume no responsibility for information accuracy.)

angelfire.com/mi/FAST (articles, recipes, and links)

foodprocessing.com (manufacturer links)

www.penny.ca/Links.htm (manufacturer's links)

www.glutenfreeinfo.com/Diet/glutenfreeinfo.htm (gluten-free manufacturer list)

www.celiac.com (Celiac Support Page)

www.finerhealth.com (gluten sensitivity information & consultation, live chat)

www.enterolab.com (gluten and yeast sensitivity testing, by mail)

http://users.aol.com/katherinez/kath2.htm#from you (Children With Milk, Egg, and Other Food Allergies)

http://dspace.dial.pipex.com/town/park/gfm11/milk2.shtml#links (dairy-free sites)

http://adelaide.net.au/~ndk/no_milk.htm (milk allergy & lactose intolerance)

http://www.panix.com/~nomilk/ (No Milk Page)

http://www.paleodiet.com Paleolithic Diet Page

http://allallergy.net/index.cfm#Food Reactions (All Allergy Net)

www.savorypalate.com (free recipes for food sensitivities)

http://www.allergykids.org/ (Allergy Kids Homepage)

http://funrsc.fairfield.edu/~jfleitas/kidsintro.html (Bandaides and Blackboards)

www.fankids.org (Food Allergy Network website for kids)

www.candida-yeast.com (Dr. William G. Crook's web site for yeast and candida)

271

Vendors (Food)

This list does not endorse any of these vendors or manufacturers, nor is it intended to include ALL of them. Verify all information before using. All produce gluten-free items, unless otherwise noted.

Allergybuyersclub.com Tapping Institute 160 Pine St., #10 Auburndale, MA 02466, 800.372.1303; 617.332.0292 - fax http://stage.acunet.net/abcsite/index.asp (consumer allergy products)	Always Natural Foods 3323 E. Patterson Road Beaver Creek, OH 45430 800.589.1709; 937.426.7464 - fax (wheat-free products)
A & A Amazing Foods, Inc.(Absersold) PO Box 3927 Citrus Heights, CA 95611 800.497.4834 (Dari-Free gluten-free milk powder)	Arrowhead Mills, Inc. Box 2059 Hereford, TX 79045 www.wholefoods.com (flours, cereals)
Authentic Foods 1850 W. 169th Street, Suite B Gardena, CA 90247 800.806.4737; 310.366.6938 - fax www.authenticfoods.com/ (garfava flour, bean flour, mixes)	Bob's Red Mill Natural Foods 5209 S.E. International Way Milwaukie, OR 97222 800.553.2258. 503.653.1339 - fax www.Bobsredmill.com (flours, grains, mixes)
'Cause You're Special Co. 815.877.6722; 603.754.0245 - fax http://www.causeyourespecial.com (all natural foods)	Cecilia's Gluten Free Grocery 800.491.2760 (orders) 775.827.0672; 775.827.5850 - fax http://www.glutenfreegrocery.com
Gluten-Free Delights, Inc. PO Box 284 Cedar Falls, IA 50613 888.403.1806 www.glutenfreedelights.com (ready-made bread)	Dietary Specialties, Inc. (MenuDirect) 865 Centennial Ave. Piscataway, NJ 08854 888.MENU123; 716.232.6168 - fax www.dietspec.com (pasta, flours, ready-made, mixes)

Vendors (continued)

Ener-G Foods, Inc. P.O. Box 84487 Seattle, WA 98124-5787 800.331.5222 206.764.3398 - fax www.ener-g.com (flours, ingredients, mixes)	Foods by George 3 King Street Mahwah, NJ 07430 201.612.9700 201.684.0334 – fax (bakery items, pasta products)
Gluten-Free Pantry PO Box 881 Glastonbury, CT 06033 800.291.8386 (orders only) 203.633.3826; 860.633.6853 - fax www.glutenfree.com (mixes, ingredients, appliances)	Glutino.com (DEROMA) 800.363.DIET (3438) 450.629.7689; 450.629.4781 – fax www.glutino.com (full line of products)
Kinnikinnick Bakery 10306-112 Street Edmonton, AB, Canada T5K 1N1 877.503.4466 780.424.2900; 780.421.0456 - fax www.kinnikinnick.com (ready-made foods, mixes)	Miss Roben's PO Box 1149 Frederick, MD 21701 800.891.0083 301.665.9580; 301.665.9584 - fax www.missroben.com (mixes, ingredients, books)
Mr. Spice Healthy Foods 850 Aquidneck Avenue Newport, RI 02842 401.848.7700; 401.848.7701 - fax (salt-free, fat-free sauces)	Nancy's Natural Foods 266 NW First Avenue, Suite A Canby, OR 97013 877. 862.4457; 301. 665. 9584 – fax nnfoods@teleport.com (mixes, flours, ingredients)
Natural Feast Corporation P. O. Box 36 Dover, MA 02030 508.984.4230; 978.785.2208 - fax www.naturalfeast.com/pie/ (ready-made pie, muffins, cakes)	Red River Milling 801 Cumberland Street Vernon, TX 76384 800.419 9614 (sorghum flour/meal/bran; mung bean flour, urid flour)

Vendors (continued)	**Vendor (Non-Food)**
Sylvan Border Farms Mendocino Gluten-Free Products, Inc. PO Box 277 Willits, CA 95490 800.297.5399; 707.459.1834 - fax http://catalog.mendofood.com/brow seGroup.cfm?item_group_id=4992 (flour, mixes)	Clan Thompson 951 Maine St. Stoneham, ME 04231 www.clanthompson.com (pocket guides for food and drugs, downloadable gluten-free food database)

Internet Support Groups

These Internet news groups provide discussions on important topics. We assume no responsibility for accuracy of information on these sites.

Celiac Disease and Wheat Sensitivities:
http://www.enabling.org/ia/celiac/#subscribe

Celiac-Diabetes:
http://www.lsoft.com/scripts/wl.exe?XH=LISTSERV.DIABETES.ORG

Cel-Kids discussion group for families of children with celiac disease:
http://maelstrom.stjohns.edu/CGI/wa.exe?SUBED1=cel-kids&A=1

No-Milk:
http://www.nomilk.com

Publications

| *Gluten-Free Living* (newsletter)
Gluten-Free Living
P.O. Box 105
Hastings-On-Hudson, NY 10706.
914.969.2018.
GFLiving@aol.com | *Sully's Living Without: A lifestyle guide for people with food and chemical sensitivities* (magazine)
P.O. Box 132
Clarendon Hills, IL 60514-0132
630.415.3378
www.livingwithout.com |

Index

276

278

About the Author

Theresa Willingham is a journalist living in Tampa, FL with her husband, Steve, and their three children. She authored human interest, travel, and medical columns and features for the Gannet newspaper, Florida Today, for over a decade. She has written for a number of publications and organizations including the Journal of the Brevard Medical Association, the Florida Institute of Technology, and Home Education Press. Her long-time interest in health issues proved valuable in dealing with her son's inability to tolerate wheat and her intensive research into food sensitivities culminated in the handbook, *The Food Allergy Field Guide: A Lifestyle Manual for Families.*

FAST, Food Allergy Survivors Together

(http://www.angelfire.com/mi/FAST/)

Contact Sheet

for Children in Daycares, Preschool, School, or with Caregivers

Information About Child:

Name: _____ _____ _____
Age:
Height: ___'___"
Weight: _____
Hair color: _____
Eye color: _____
Male ☐ Female☐
See picture at right
Child reacts to allergens (typically) in this way: _____
Page added (child's reactions to food, etc.) ☐
_____
_____

Child's photo here

Allergies
Dairy☐ Eggs ☐ Wheat ☐ Potato☐ Peanuts☐ Tree nuts☐ Fish ☐Shellfish ☐Soy☐Other ☐
_____, _____, _____,
Please note that these allergens can go by different names. For example, albumin can mean "eggs," "lactose" is milk. Alternate names for the above allergens include: _____, _____, _____, _____, _____, _____,
_____, _____, _____
Safe foods: _____, _____, _____, _____, _____, _____, _____,
_____, _____, _____
☐ Being touched/ exposed to an allergen (not just ingesting) can cause an allergic reaction in _____.
☐ Page added (safe foods included with child, additional allergens, etc.)

Contact Information

Father's name: _____
Work phone: _____-_____
Mother's name: _____
Work phone: _____-_____
Parents' home phone number: _____-_____
Parents' beeper, cell phone, or other way of contacting: _____
Neighbor's home work number: ___-_____ (Name: _____)
Friend's home work number: ___-_____ (Name: _____)
Friend's home work number: ___-_____ (Name: _____)
Friend's home work number: ___-_____ (Name: _____)
Page added (who to contact) ☐

Treatment if Exposed

Number, in order, of which to contact first.
Parent (numbers listed above) ☐
Family doctor's number: ____-_____
Pediatrician's number: ____-_____
Hospital: ____-_____
Allergist's number: ____-_____
911
Use EpiPen
(Instructions {where stored, how to administer, etc.}: _____
_____
_____
_____)
Page added (treatment information) ☐
Parents can fill out this sheet with the help and input of their allergist, and append any needed information.